Get Through

MRCPCH Part 2: Data Interpretation Questions

Second E

Nagi Giumm

FRCPCH, CASLA

Consultant Paedi

Honorary Consu

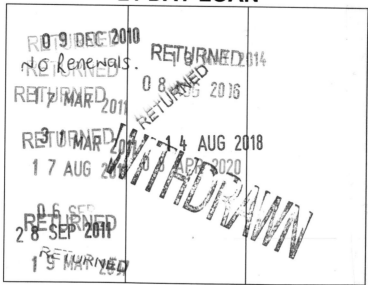

© 2008 Royal Society of Medicine Ltd

Published by the Royal Society of Medicine Press Ltd
1 Wimpole Street, London W1G 0AE, UK
Tel: +44 (0)20 7290 2921
Fax: +44 (0)20 7290 2929
E-mail: publishing@rsmpress.co.uk

British Library Cataloguing in Publication Data
A catalogue record for this book is available from the British Library

ISBN: 978-1-85315-731-8

Distribution in Europe and Rest of World:

Marston Book Services Ltd
PO Box 269
Abingdon
Oxon OX14 4YN, UK
Tel: +44 (0)1235 465500
Fax: +44 (0)1235 465555
Email: direct.order@marston.co.uk

Distribution in the USA and Canada:

Royal Society of Medicine Press Ltd
c/o BookMasters Inc
30 Amberwood Parkway
Ashland, OH 44805, USA
Tel: +1 800 247 6553/ +1 800 266 5564
Fax: +1 410 281 6883
Email: order@bookmasters.com

Distribution in Australia and New Zealand:

Elsevier Australia
30–52 Smidmore Street
Marrickville NSW 2204, Australia
Tel: +61 2 9517 8999
Fax: +61 2 9517 2249
Email: service@elsevier.com.au

Typeset by Phoenix Photosetting, Chatham, Kent
Printed in the UK by Bell & Bain, Glasgow

Contents

Dedication

To Lobna, Iman, Nadia, Yasmine and Abdulhakim

'I am not sure what I want to be. I think I would like to be a doctor to help people not get diseases and to save people's lives.

Doctors are much respected for what they do. They work very hard in hospital and they study very hard to become doctors. They try raising money for charity and they work in busy hospitals.

Some doctors perform operations and they can make people walk again after accidents. They also can help you if you have a broken arm or leg.'

Nadia Barakat

Preface

This book is designed for postgraduate candidates taking the MRCPCH Part 2 clinical exams in the UK and Ireland. It can also be used as reference to many clinical cases when teaching clinical paediatric medicine to undergraduate or postgraduate students. It offers an easily accessible and very comprehensive review of some of the most common cases and a few of the rare ones that one may encounter. All cases are real cases, which have been collected from personal experience while I was working as a consultant in paediatrics over the past seven years.

This book is different from the first edition, *100 Data Interpretation Questions in Paediatrics for MRCPCH/MRCP*, which was published in 1999, in that it has four different question styles: best of list, n from many, extended matching questions, and questions to which you have to respond with a written answer. It covers all paediatric specialties, with a little bit more on paediatric neurology as this area is a special interest of mine. The explanation and discussion of the topics is not very long, and most of the time I have tried to use my personal experience as well as covering key information about the topic of the case. I have tried to include the pathophysiology in as many cases as possible, as I find it most exciting and helpful to understand the illness. There are a few unusual cases, such as Aicardi syndrome, which may be described to the candidate as 'a failure to thrive'.

The book has been divided into ten sections or 'papers', each of which consists of ten case presentations and between one and four questions relating to each case; answers are given at the end of each paper. Always try to write down on paper your answer to the questions before going on to read the answers and explanation.

This book is a practical study aid for both the written and clinical MRCPCH examinations, giving the reader a variety of different styles of questions with which to test their knowledge. Some of the answers are helpful for paediatricians to use as guidelines for the investigation of many cases. Medical students will learn about clinical paediatrics if they read the cases and their explanations.

As my area of special interest is medical education, I have recently completed my degree in medical education from Imperial College, London (CASLAT). I tried to make this book as clinically oriented as possible and to use the problem-based learning method of getting clinical scenarios related to day-to-day work as well as teaching. I hope you enjoy using this book.

NAGI GIUMMA BARAKAT

Acknowledgements

Special thanks are due to my wife and my children, from whom I took valuable time to complete this book, and I hope that one day they may forgive me. I also thank Mrs Lynn Frame, who checked and edited this book before sending it to the RSM. The team at the RSM Press were very patient with me even when the due date for transmittal of the manuscript was not met. I would like to thank Professor J Aicardi, Professor C Hughs, Dr GM Fenichel and Dr RJ Postlethwaite and their publishers (MacKeith Press, Butterworth Heinemann and WB Saunders) for allowing me to use material from their books and journal articles.

References and further reading

Aicardi J (1998) *Diseases of the Nervous System in Childhood*, 2nd edn. Cambridge: MacKeith Press.

Bailey W, Freidenberg GR, James HE et al (1990) Prenatal diagnosis of a craniopharyngioma using ultrasonography. *Prenat Diagn* 10: 623–9.

Bardella IJ (1999) Pediatric advanced life support: a review of the AHA recommendations. *Am Fam Physician* 60: 1743–50 [Erratum 2000; 61: 2014].

Driscoll DA, Budarf ML, Emanuel BS (1992) A genetic etiology for DiGeorge syndrome: consistent deletions and microdeletions of 22q11. *Am J Hum Genet* 50: 924–33.

Fenichel GM (2005) *Clinical Pediatric Neurology: A Signs and Symptoms Approach*, 5th edn. London: WB Saunders.

Havel RJ, Kane JP (2001) Structure and metabolism of plasma lipoproteins. In: Scriver CR, Beaudet AL, Valle D et al, eds. *The Metabolic and Molecular Bases of Inherited Disease*, 8th edn. New York: McGraw-Hill: 2705–16.

Hodson EM, Willis NS, Craig JC (2001) Non-corticosteroid treatment for nephritic syndrome in children. *Cochrane Database Syst Rev* (4): CD002290.

Hoffmann HJ, Hendrick EB, Humphreys RP et al (1977) Management of craniopharyngiomas in children. *J Neurosurg* 47: 218–27.

Lim J, McKean M (2001) Adenotonsillectomy for obstructive sleep apnoea in children. *Cochrane Database Syst Rev* (3): CD003136.

McIntosh N, Helms P, Smyth R, eds (2003) *Forfar and Arneil's Textbook of Paediatrics*, 6th edn. Edinburgh: Churchill Livingstone.

NICE (2007) Urinary Tract Infection in Children: Diagnosis, Treatment and Long-Term Management. NICE Clinical Guideline 54, August 2007. National Institute for Health and Clinical Excellence. www.nice.org.uk/nicemedia/pdf/CG54NICEguideline.pdf.

Puckett RM, Offringa M (2000) Prophylactic vitamin K for vitamin K deficiency bleeding in neonates. *Cochrane Database Syst Rev* (4): CD002776.

Rosenblum ND, Winter HS (1987) Steroid effects on the course of abdominal pain in children with Henoch–Schönlein purpura. *Paediatrics* 79: 1018–21.

Webb NJA, Postlethwaite RJ (2003) *Clinical Paediatric Nephrology*, 3rd edn. Oxford: Oxford University Press.

Other resources include the journals *Archives of Disease in Childhood*, *Current Paediatrics* and the *European Journal of Paediatric Neurology* (among others) and the eMedicine website www.emedicine.com.

Abbreviations

17–OHP	17–Hydroxyprogesterone
25(OH)D	25–Hydroxyvitamin D
AA	Amino acids
AAFB	Alcohol- and acid-fast bacilli
ABG	Arterial blood gas
ACTH	Adrenocorticotropic hormone
ADH	Antidiuretic hormone
AGN	Acute glomerulonephritis
AIDS	Acquired immune deficiency syndrome
Alb	Albumin
aGT	α-glutamic transaminase
ALP	Alkaline phosphatase
ALT	Alanine aminotransferase
ANA	Antinuclear antibodies
AO	Aorta
APTT	Activated partial thromboplastin time
AR	Autosomal recessive
ASD	Atrial septal defect
ASOT	Anti-streptolysin-O-titres
AST	Aspartate aminotransferase
AXR	Abdominal X-ray
BCG	Bacillus Calmette–Guérin
BE	Base excess
Bili	Bilirubin
BMD	Bone metabolic disease
BPD	Broncho-pulmonary dysplasia
BSAER	Brainstem auditory evoked response
BT	Bleeding time
C3	Complement
Ca	Calcium
CAH	Congenital adrenal hyperplasia
CF	Cystic fibrosis
CH50	Cytochrome 50
CHO	Carbohydrate
CI	Confidence interval
CK	Creatine kinase
Cl	Chloride
CMV	Cytomegalovirus
CNS	Central nervous system
CO_2	Carbon dioxide
CPAP	Continuous positive airway pressure
Cr	Creatinine
CRP	C-reactive protein
CT	Computed tomography
CXR	Chest X-ray
DCT	Direct Coombs test
DHEA	Dehydroepiandrosterone
DKA	Diabetic ketoacidosis

DMD	Duchenne muscular dystrophy
DMSA	Dimercaptosuccinic acid
DNA	Deoxyribonucleic acid
D/S	Diastolic/systolic
DTPA	Diethylene triamine pentaacetic acid
EBV	Epstein–Barr virus
Echo	Echocardiograph
EEG	Electroencephalogram
ELSCS	Elective lower segmental caesarean section
EMG	Electromyography
ERCP	Endoscopic retrograde cholangiopancreatography
ERG	Electro-retinography
ESR	Erythrocyte sedimentation rate
ETT	Endotracheal tube
FA	Fanconi anaemia
FBC	Full blood count
FEF	Forced expiration flow
FEV_1	Forced expiratory volume in 1 second
Fib	Fibrinogen
FSH	Follicle-stimulating hormone
FVC	Forced vital capacity
FVII	Factor VII
FVIII	Factor VIII
FVIIIC	Coagulation factor VIII
G6PD	Glucose-6-phosphate dehydrogenase
GBS	Guillain–Barré syndrome
GFR	Glomerular filtration rate
GH	Growth hormone
GHI	Growth hormone insufficiency
GHD	Growth hormone deficiency
GIT	Gastrointestinal tract
Glc	Glucose
GN	Glomerulonephritis
GnRH	Gonadotropin-releasing hormone
GOR	Gastro-oesophageal reflux
GORD	Gastro-oesophageal reflux disease
GVHD	Graft versus host disease
Hb	Haemoglobin
HbF	Fetal haemoglobin
HCO^{-3}	Bicarbonate
Hct	Haematocrit
HIV	Human immunodeficiency virus
HMD	Hyaline membrane disease
HR	Heart rate
HSV	Herpes simplex virus
HUS	Haemolytic uraemic syndrome
HVA	Homovanillic acid
IBD	Irritable bowel disease
Ig	Immunoglobulin
IGF	Insulin-like growth factor
INR	International Normalized Ratio
IRT	Immunoreactive trypsin

iT	Inspiratory time
ITP	Idiopathic thrombocytopenic purpura
ITT	Insulin tolerance test
IUGR	Intrauterine growth restriction
IVC	Inferior vena cava
IVH	Intraventricular haemorrhage
IVIG	Intravenous immunoglobulin
IVU	Intravenous urogram
K	Potassium
KUB	Kidney, ureters and bladder
LA	Left atrium
LBBB	Left bundle branch block
LFT	Liver function test
LH	Luteinizing hormone
LHRH	Luteinizing hormone-releasing hormone
LP	Lumbar puncture
LV	Left ventricle
MAG3	Mercapto acetyl triglycine
MAP	Mean arterial pressure
MCHC	Mean corpuscular haemoglobin concentration
MCUG	Micturating cystourethrogram
MCV	Mean corpuscular volume
MELAS	Mitochondrial encephalopathy, lactic acidosis and stroke-like episodes
Mg	Magnesium
MIBG	*m*-Iodobenzylguanidine
MRA	Magnetic resonance angiography
MRI	Magnetic resonance imaging
MS	Multiple sclerosis
MSU	Midstream urine
Na	Sodium
NADP(H)	Nicotinamide adenine dinucleotide phosphate (reduced)
NBT	Nitroblue tetrazolium test
NCPAP	Nasal continuous positive airway pressure
NCS	Nerve conduction study
NEC	Necrotizing enterocolitis
NH_4	Ammonium
NPA	Naso-pharyngeal aspirate
NS	Normal saline
NSAID	Non-steroidal anti-inflammatory drug
O_2	Oxygen
OFC	Occipitofrontal circumference
P	Phosphorus
PA	Pulmonary artery
Pb	Lead
P_{CO_2}	Carbon dioxide tension
PCP	*Pneumocystis jiroveci (carinii)* pneumonia
PCR	Polymerase chain reaction
PCV	Packed cell volume
PDA	Patent ductus arteriosus
PEEP	Peak end-expiratory pressure
PEF	Peak expiratory flow

PEFR	Peak expiratory flow rate
pH	Logarithmic hydrogen ion concentration
PHA	Phytohaemoagglutinin
PHH	Post-haemorrhagic hydrocephalus
PICU	Paediatric intensive care unit
PIP	Peak inspiratory pressure
Plt	Platelets
Po_2	Oxygen tension
PO_4	Phosphate
PT	Prothrombin time
PTT	Partial thromboplastin time
PV	Pulmonary vein
RA	Right atrium
RAST	Radioallergosorbent test
RCoF	Ristocetin cofactor
RBBB	Right bundle branch block
RBC	Red blood cells
Ret	Reticulocytes
RNA	Ribonucleic acid
RR	Respiratory rate
RS	Reye syndrome
RTA	Renal tubular acidosis
RV	Right ventricle
Sao_2	Oxygen saturation
SIADH	Syndrome of inappropriate ADH secretion
SLE	Systemic lupus erythematosus
SSRI	Selective serotonin re-uptake inhibitor
SVC	Superior vena cava
SVT	Supraventricular tachycardia
SXR	Skull X-ray
T_4	Thyroxine
TAPVD	Total anomalous pulmonary venous drainage
TAR	Thrombocytopenia-absent radius
TB	Tuberculosis
TFT	Thyroid function test
TGA	Transposition of the great arteries
TLC	Total lung capacity
TPN	Total parenteral nutrition
TRH	Thyroid-releasing hormone
TSH	Thyroid-stimulating hormone
TT	Thrombin time
TV	Tidal volume
U	Urea
UAC	Umbilical artery catheter
U&E	Urea and electrolytes
UCD	Urea cycle disorder
U:P	Urine:plasma
URTI	Upper respiratory tract infection
US	Ultrasound
UTI	Urinary tract infection
UVC	Umbilical venous catheter
VC	Vital capacity

VLCFA	Very long-chain fatty acids
VEP	Visual evoked potentials
VMA	Vanillylmandelic acid
VSD	Ventricular septal defect
VUR	Vesico-ureteric reflux
vWD	von Willebrand disease
vWF	von Willebrand factor
vWF:Ag	von Willebrand factor antigen
WAS	Wiskott–Aldrich syndrome
WCC	White cell count (N, neutrophils; L, lymphocytes; E, eosinophils; M, monocytes)

Case 1

A 15-year-old girl is referred with menorrhagia and anaemia. She suffers frequent bruises during basketball games. Her mother is concerned about excessive loss of blood during her period.

Results reveal:

Hb	9.1 g/dl
MCV	85 fl
WCC	$7.2 \times 10^9/l$
MCHC	32 g/dl
Plt	$350 \times 10^9/l$
PT	14 s (normal 14 s)
APTT	60 s (normal 40 s)

1. **What is the most likely diagnosis?**
   a. Haemophilia B
   b. Leukaemia
   c. Fanconi anaemia
   d. Aplastic anaemia
   e. Von Willebrand disease

2. **What other four investigations are indicated?**
   a. FVIIIC assay
   b. Platelet aggregation with ristocetin
   c. vWF:Ag assay
   d. Family study
   e. Bone marrow aspiration
   f. Factor X assay

3. **What is the inheritance of this condition?**
   a. Sporadic
   b. Autosomal recessive
   c. Autosomal dominant
   d. X-linked recessive
   e. None of the above

Case 2

This is a sleep EEG of a 9-year-old girl referred to the Outpatients Department with a history of generalized seizures and abnormal movement of the mouth during the seizure. She has had three attacks – all of them at night.

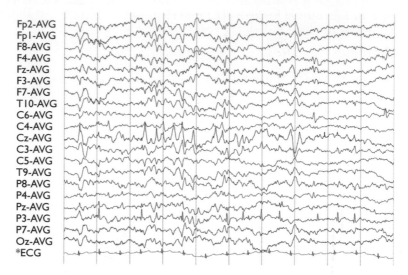

1. **What is the diagnosis?**
   a. Juvenile myoclonic epilepsy (JME)
   b. Childhood absence epilepsy syndrome (CAES)
   c. Landau–Kleffner syndrome
   d. Benign Rolandic epilepsy of childhood
   e. Electrical status epilepticus during sleep (ESES)

2. **What further test can be done?**
   a. MRI scan
   b. Video telemetry over 48 hours
   c. Repeat EEG
   d. Magnetic EEG
   e. None of the above

3. **What is the treatment?**
   a. Clobazam
   b. Sodium valproate
   c. Levetiracetam
   d. Carbamazepine
   e. None of the above

Case 3

This is a family tree with a diagnosis of Duchenne muscular dystrophy.

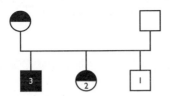

1. What is the mode of inheritance?
2. What is the risk of being affected or a carrier for:
    1.
    2.
    3.

Case 4

A 14-year-old girl is admitted with a history of abdominal pain. There is tenderness over the right upper quadrant. A splenectomy was performed at the age of 10 years.

Hb	13.1 g/dl
WCC	$7 \times 10^9/l$
Plt	$210 \times 10^9/l$
Blood film	Spherocytes and anisocytosis, Howell–Jolly bodies

1. What is the most likely cause of her abdominal pain?
    a. Bowel obstruction
    b. Ovarian cyst
    c. Renal hydronephrosis
    d. Gallbladder stones
    e. Constipation

2. What is the single most useful investigation?
    a. ERCP
    b. Upper GIT endoscopy
    c. Abdominal ultrasound
    d. Abdominal MRI scan
    e. Barium swallow and follow-through

Case 5

A 6-month-old male infant presents with watery diarrhoea and nappy rash, which has been present for the last 2 weeks. The boy was born by normal vaginal delivery and weighed 3.2 kg. The health visitor is concerned that he is failing to thrive. Three uncles died early in childhood.

Hb	13 g/dl
Plt	443×10^9/l
WCC	4.3×10^9/l (N 2.9, L 0.9, M 0.3)
CD3	4%
CD4	3%
CD8	3% (all are low)
PHA	No response
IgG	115 g/l
IgA	7 g/l
IgM	14 g/l
Mg	0.8 mmol/l
Ca	1.7 mmol/l
PO$_4$	1.2 mmol/l
CXR	Thymic tissue absent

1. **What is the most likely diagnosis?**
   a. Severe combined immune deficiency
   b. Autoimmune deficiency syndrome
   c. DiGeorge syndrome
   d. Chronic granulomatous disease
   e. Wiskott–Aldrich syndrome

2. **What is the inheritance?**
   a. Sporadic
   b. AD
   c. X-linked recessive
   d. AR
   e. X-linked dominant
   f. Unknown

3. **Name one supportive diagnostic investigation.**
   a. Bone marrow aspiration
   b. Skin biopsy
   c. Thymus scan
   d. Fluorescent in situ hybridization chromosomal analysis (FISH 22)
   e. None of the above

Case 6

A boy can draw a square and mimic a bridge with cubes. He can only say 20 single words and can name three colours.

1. **What is his age?**

2. **What further management would be required for his problem?**

Case 7

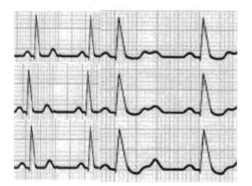

This is an ECG for a 4-year-old child who presented with DKA and was treated with IV insulin and normal saline (maintenance + 7% deficit). Blood was taken after 18 hours of treatment.

Na	134 mmol/l
pH	7.29
K	2.3 mmol/l
CO_2	3.9 kPa
ESR	25 mm/h
BE	−6.5
CXR	Normal
LFT and clotting	Normal

1. What are the abnormalities on ECG?

2. What is the diagnosis?

Case 8

A 14-year-old girl with known type 1 diabetes over the last 9 years has a urine test that showed albumin of 30 µg/min (normal <20 µg/min). She is on twice daily insulin of M30/70.

Na	140 mmol/l
HbA_{1c}	11.4%
K	4.6 mmol/l
U	5 mmol/l
Cr	65 mmol/l
LFT and clotting	Normal

1. What is the most likely diagnosis?

2. Name one test that may help to establish the diagnosis.

Case 9

An 18-month-old presents with vomiting, failure to thrive and excessive drinking

Urine	pH<5.3
Glycosuria /generalized aminoaciduria/proteinuria	
Na	136 mmol/l
HCO^{-3}	13 mmol/l
K	3.3 mmol/l
PO_4	0.9 mmol/l
AXR	Nephrocalcinosis
LFT and clotting	Normal

1. What is the diagnosis?

2. What is the underlying problem?

Case 10

A 5-day-old baby presents with vomiting and lethargy and has not passed urine over the last 18 hours. His mother is known to have had diabetes since the age of 10 years. There is a left renal mass.

Na	144 mmol/l
K	5.3 mmol/l
U	7.8 mm/h
Cr	125 mmol/l
Hb	16.3 g/dl
Plt	60×10^9/l
LFT and clotting	Normal
Urine:	
Protein	+++
RBC	+++

1. What is the most likely diagnosis?
   a. Acute tubular necrosis
   b. Sepsis
   c. Left renal vein thrombosis
   d. Wilms tumour
   e. Hydronephrosis

2. What other two investigations will you carry out?
   a. Renal ultrasound
   b. Renal venography
   c. Abdominal CT scan
   d. IVU
   e. MAG3 scan

Case 1

1. Von Willebrand disease
2. FVIIIC assay, uWF:Ag assay, platelet aggregation with ristocetin, family study
3. Autosomal dominant

Von Willebrand disease (vWD)

vWD is usually inherited as an autosomal dominant trait. It is caused by underproduction or dysfunction of von Willebrand factor (vWF). There are three types of vWD: in type 1 there is a partial quantitative deficiency in vWF; in type 2 a variety of functional and structural defects (which distinguish four subtypes: 2A, 2B, 2M and 2N), and in type 3 a near total deficiency.

	Type I	Type II	Type III
Inheritance	Autosomal dominant	Autosomal dominant	Autosomal recessive
FVIIIC activity	Mildly decreased	Normal or decreased[a]	Greatly decreased
vWF level	Decreased	Normal or decreased[a]	Greatly decreased or absent
vWF function	Normal	Abnormal	Greatly decreased or absent
vWF structure	Normal	Normal or abnormal[a]	Normal (when present)
Platelet function	Abnormal	Abnormal	Abnormal

[a]Depending on subtype.

On presentation, there is usually a history of prolonged nasal and gum bleeding, and prolonged oozing. PT is in the normal range, but APTT is increased in some vWD types.

Case 2

1. Centro-temporal spike and waves (benign Rolandic epilepsy of childhood)
2. None
3. None

Benign Rolandic seizures

The EEG shows bilateral centro-temporal spikes during sleep.

This is one of the most common forms of epilepsy in childhood, being found in 15–20% of young patients with epilepsy. The age of onset ranges from 3 to 13 years. About 40% of close relatives have been found to have a history of febrile convulsion, partial or generalized seizures, or epileptic discharges in the EEG of a focal or generalized nature. These include slow, dysphasic, high-voltage, centro-temporal spikes, activated by sleep. Neuroimaging is normal.

Clinical features

The typical presentation occurs either upon awakening or during sleep; the child comes to its parents, fully conscious but unable to speak, pointing to its mouth, which is drawn to one side, with saliva oozing from one corner; this is often followed by hemifacial twitching. The whole episode lasts for one or two minutes. The other type of nocturnal seizure is characterized by vocal noises with grunting and gurgling sounds coming from the child's mouth, which is drawn to one side and drooling. The patient usually loses consciousness with this type of seizure, and the seizure may become generalized. The third type of presentation is with secondary generalized tonic/clonic seizures. These occur during sleep and last from a few minutes to 30 minutes; they may be followed by a Todd paralysis (Aicardi 1998). The somatosensory aura is probably common, but children rarely report it as the seizures always occur during the night. The seizures usually appear in the first decade of life and disappear in the second. There is no cerebral lesion and the affected child is usually healthy.

Treatment

Treatment is not required unless the episodes happen during the daytime, are too frequent or there is parental concern. Carbamezapine should be tried first. If there is no response then clobazam, sodium valproate or lamotrigine should be tried. Approximately 80% of seizures respond to anticonvulsant therapy. The prognosis is excellent and the EEGs normalize within a few years of the disappearance of the seizures.

Case 3

1. X-linked recessive
2.
    1. Male is affected
    2. Female is a carrier
    3. Male is healthy

The daughters of an affected male will all be carriers of an X-linked recessive gene and affected by an X-linked dominant one.

A woman who is a carrier will have 1 in 2 affected sons; half of her daughters will be carriers if the disease is autosomal recessive, and all of her daughters will be affected if the disease is X-linked dominant.

Case 4

1. Gallbladder stones
2. Abdominal ultrasound

Gallstones in children

There are different types of gallstones, in the form of cholesterol, bile pigment, calcium and inorganic matrix. About 70% are formed from bile pigment, and these are radio-opaque. Cholesterol is a constituent of 15–20% of gallstones and is radiolucent. Gallstones may present as recurrent abdominal pain and/or acute cholecystitis. Ultrasound is the diagnostic investigation of choice.

Causes and precipitating factors

These include obesity, sickle cell disease, ileal resection and disease, cystic fibrosis, prolonged parenteral nutrition, chemotherapy for childhood cancer, and abdominal surgery.

The most common type of gallstones associated with spherocytosis are those formed by pigmentary bilirubin. They may be formed as early as 4–5 years of age; 50% of splenectomized patients will develop pigmentary gall stones, which are usually asymptomatic. The osmotic fragility test is not done routinely in many hospitals.

Spherocytes undergo lysis more readily than biconcave red blood cells in a hypotonic solution. This tendency becomes greater if the cells are deprived of glucose over 24 hours and incubated at 37 °C. A specific protein abnormality can also be established in 80% of patients with spherocytosis by red cell membrane protein analysis using gel electrophoresis.

Case 5

1. DiGeorge syndrome
2. Unknown
3. Fluorescent in situ hybridization chromosomal analysis (FISH 22)

DiGeorge syndrome

The data suggest cell-mediated immune deficiency with low lymphocytes, low CDs and absence of the thymus gland. There is also a history of failure to thrive and recurrent chest infection.

Hypocalcaemia due to hypoparathyroidism is another feature. All of these are suggestive of DiGeorge syndrome.

Clinical features

These include hypoparathyroidism with convulsions and tetany due to hypocalcaemia. Absence of the thymus is associated with recurrent infections because of impaired cell-mediated immunity.

Other features include:

- Palatal abnormalities (e.g. cleft lip and/or palate)
- Feeding difficulties
- Conotruncal heart defects (e.g. tetralogy of Fallot, interrupted aortic arch, ventricular septal defects, vascular rings)

- Hearing loss or abnormal ear examinations
- Genitourinary anomalies (absent or malformed kidney)
- Microcephaly (small head)
- Mental retardation (usually borderline to mild)
- IQs are generally in the 70–90 range
- Psychiatric disorders in adults (e.g. schizophrenia, bipolar disorder)
- Severe immunologic dysfunction (an immune system which does not work properly due to abnormal T-cells, causing frequent infections).

Pathophysiology

DiGeorge syndrome is the result of a developmental defect of the third and fourth pharyngeal pouches and the fourth branchial arch. There is a partial monosomy of the proximal long arm of chromosome 22 in 30%, and deletion in 88% as demonstrated by FISH studies (Driscoll et al 1992). The heterogeneity of this syndrome means that it can be partial rather than the full picture.

Management

Treatment of immune deficiency has been successfully achieved using fetal thymus implants or bone marrow transplants (McIntosh et al 2003).

Case 6

1. Age is 4 years.
2. Speech therapy referral, educational authority referral.

Speech delay

Speech delay can be caused by anatomical problems with the vocal cords, brain trauma or hearing loss, or difficulties with the processing of speech (mental retardation and developmental language disorders). The two main types of speech delay are expressive delay, which is the inability to generate speech, and receptive delay, the inability to decode or understand the speech of others. Some children can have a delay that is a mix of both types (mixed expressive/receptive delay).

Most children with speech delay have a developmental language problem. In some it is constitutional and in others related to developmental disorders such as autism.

It is very important to know normal speech milestones before diagnosing delay in speech. Testing of hearing must be done before making the final diagnosis.

Age of the child	What he/she should achieve in speech
1–6 months	Coos in response to voice
6–9 months	Babbling
10–11 months	Imitation of sounds; says 'mama/dada' without meaning
12 months	Says 'mama/dada' with meaning; often imitates two- and three-syllable words

13–15 months	Vocabulary of 4–7 words in addition to jargon; <20% of speech understood by strangers
16–18 months	Vocabulary of 10 words; some echolalia and extensive jargon; 20–25% of speech understood by strangers
19–21 months	Vocabulary of 20 words; 50% of speech understood by strangers
22–24 months	Vocabulary >50 words; two-word phrases; dropping out of jargon; 60–70% of speech understood by strangers
2–2½ years	Vocabulary of 400 words, including names; 2–3 word phrases; use of pronouns; diminishing echolalia; 75% of speech understood by strangers
2½–3 years	Use of plurals and past tense; knows age and sex; counts three objects correctly; 3–5 words per sentence; 80–90% of speech understood by strangers
3–4 years	Three to six words per sentence; asks questions, converses, relates experiences, tells stories; almost all speech understood by strangers
4–5 years	Six to eight words per sentence; names four colours; counts 10 pennies correctly

Case 7

1. ST-segment depression
   Prolonged QT interval
   Decreased T wave
2. Hypokalaemia

ECG changes associated with biochemical disturbances of hypokalaemia

The ECG can be described as follows: sinus bradycardia and electrocardiographic (ECG) signs of hypokalaemia (U waves in leads II, V_2, V_3 and V_4, progressive flattening of T waves and depression of ST segment) may appear when the serum potassium falls below normal. Prolongation of the PR and QT intervals and T-wave flattening are associated with prominent U waves.

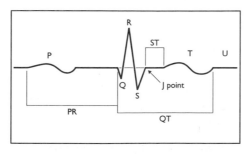

Hypokalaemia:

a. Prolonged QT interval
b. ST-segment depression
c. T-wave flattening
d. Appearance of U wave
e. Ventricular dysrhythmia

ECG abnormalities associated with hyperkalaemia are:

a. Appearance of tall, pointed, narrow T waves
b. Decreased P-wave amplitude, decreased R-wave height, widening of QRS complexes, ST-segment changes (elevation/depression), hemi-block (especially left anterior) and first-degree heart block
c. Advanced intraventricular block (very wide QRS with RBBB, LBBB, bi- or tri-fascicular blocks) and ventricular ectopics
d. Absent P waves; very broad, bizarre QRS complexes; AV block; VT, VF or ventricular asystole.

Hypocalcaemia and hypomagnesaemia ECG changes are prolongation of the QTc interval because of lengthening of the ST segment, and decreased ST voltage in 50% of patients. Hypocalcaemia generally does not cause T-wave changes, because it does not affect phase 3 of the action potential.

In hypercalcaemia, QT-interval shortening is common, and, in some cases, the PR interval is prolonged. At very high levels, the QRS interval may lengthen, T waves may flatten or invert, and a variable degree of heart block may develop.

In hypernatraemia and hyponatraemia, there are no significant ECG changes.

Case 8

1. Microalbuminuria
2. Renal biopsy

Complications associated with type 1 diabetes:

- Hypoglycaemia
- DKA
- Hypercholesterolaemia
- Visual impairment
- Renal failure
- Stroke
- Blindness
- Myocardial infarction
- Amputation

The changes in the kidneys and other organs such as retina, brain, and peripheral nerves are related to microvascular disease. It is a form of hyaline arteriosclerosis, characterized by wall thickening of the small arterioles and large capillaries. The wall thickening leads to diabetic nephropathy, which is characterized by proteinuria, glomerular hyalinization (Kimmelstiel–Wilson syndrome) and chronic renal failure.

Case 9

1. Fanconi syndrome
2. Distal RTA
   Primary hyperparathyroidism
   Medullary sponge kidney

Nephrocalcinosis

Nephrocalcinosis can be either micro- or macroscopic. It is caused by hypercalcaemia. The patient can present with polydipsia and polyuria. There is glycosuria, aminoaciduria and proteinuria, and more than half of patients are hypertensive. Other causes include hypervitaminosis D, idiopathic hypercalciuria, hypophosphataemia, renal papillary necrosis, progressive osteoporosis, and chronic hypokalaemic states, such as Bartter syndrome, primary hyperaldosteronism, Liddle syndrome and 11β-hydroxylase deficiency.

Case 10

1. Left renal vein thrombosis
2. Renal venography
   Renal ultrasound

Renal vein thrombosis

In the newborn period, renal vein thrombosis may complicate sepsis or dehydration. It may be observed in an infant of a diabetic mother; may be associated with umbilical vein catheterization; or may result from any condition that produces a hypercoagulable state (e.g. clotting factor deficiency, systemic lupus erythematosus or thrombocytosis). Renal vein thrombosis is less common in older children and adolescents. It may develop following trauma or without any apparent predisposing factors. Spontaneous renal vein thrombosis has been associated with membranous glomerulonephropathy. Nephrotic syndrome may either cause or result from renal vein thrombosis. Renal vein thrombosis in newborns is generally characterized by the sudden development of an abdominal mass. If the thrombosis is bilateral, oliguria may be present; urine output may be normal with a unilateral thrombus. In older children, flank pain, sometimes with a palpable mass, is a common presentation. Ultrasound and Doppler scan may help in diagnosis, but renal venography will help in diagnosing renal vein thrombosis in children. Treatment is usually conservative, and there is a debate about using anticoagulants. The majority will recover if the cause is treated successfully. A few children may need dialysis for a short period.

Case 11

A 3-year-old child presents with swelling of his face and abdomen. He is passing dark urine.

Na	134 mmol/l
K	4.3 mmol/l
U	6.8 mm/h
Cr	95 mmol/l
Hb	11.3 g/dl
Plt	160×10^9
C3	Reduced
LFT and clotting	Normal
Urine:	
Protein	+
RBC	+++
Red cell casts	

1. **What is the most likely diagnosis?**
   a. Haemolytic uraemic syndrome
   b. Acute renal failure
   c. Nephrotic syndrome
   d. Acute glomurulonephritis
   e. Capillary leak syndrome

2. **What bedside tests can be done?**
   a. Fundus examination
   b. Measuring blood pressure
   c. ECG
   d. Daily weight
   e. None of the above

Case 12

A 3-year-old girl presents with vomiting and delirium and is confused. She has just recovered from chickenpox.

ALP	1300 mmol/l
ALT	130 mmol/l
Bilirubin	7 mmol/l
Albumin	70 mmol/l
Hb	16.3 g/dl
Glucose	2.1 mmol/l
Amylase	220 mmol/l
Na	137 mmol/l
K	3.9 mmol/l
U	4.6 mmol/l
Plt	190×10^9/l
Ammonia	200 mmol/l

1. **What is the most likely diagnosis?**
    a. Urea cycle defect
    b. Reye syndrome
    c. Primary carnitine deficiency
    d. Mitochondrial cytopathy
    e. None of the above

2. **What further two tests would you carry out?**
    a. Liver biopsy
    b. EEG
    c. MRI brain
    d. White cell enzymes
    e. Clotting screen
    f. LP

Case 13

A 7-year-old girl presents with lethargy, loss of weight and excessive drinking. Her weight is 22 kg.

Na	132 mmol/l
K	5.3 mmol/l
U	7.8 mm/h
Cr	80 mmol/l
Hb	15.3 g/dl
Plt	300×10^9/l
pH	7.23
P_{CO_2}	2.5
HCO^{-3}	13
WCC	17×10^9/l (N 70%)
BE	−17
CRP	10 mg/l
LFT and clotting	Normal
Urine:	
Protein	0
RBC	0
Glucose	+++
Ketones	+++

1. **What is the most likely diagnosis?**
    a. Septicaemia
    b. SIADH
    c. DKA
    d. Inborn error of metabolism
    e. None of the above

2. **What is your initial management? (Choose four)**
    a. IV antibiotics
    b. IV insulin
    c. IV 0.9% NaCl (240 ml)
    d. IV 0.9% NaCl with 5% glucose (3750 ml)
    e. IV 0.45% NaCl with 5% glucose (3750 ml)

f.   KCl (10 mmol for each litre of fluid)
g.   KCl (20 mmol for each litre of fluid)
h.   Bladder catheterization

Case 14

A 4-year-old girl who has just returned from India presents with tachypnoea, chest pain and mild fever.

Na	128 mmol/l
K	4.3 mmol/l
U	6.8 mm/h
Cr	80 mmol/l
Hb	12.3 g/dl
Plt	400×10^9/l
pH	7.33
HCO^{-3}	18
WCC	22×10^9/l (N 70%)
P_{CO_2}	4.5
BE	0.0
CRP	420
Urine:	
Na	40 mmol/l (20 mmol/l)
RBCs	0
Glucose	0
Ketones	+

1.   **What is the diagnosis from the biochemical results?**
     a.   Severe dehydration
     b.   Acute renal failure
     c.   Pre-renal failure
     d.   SIADH
     e.   None of the above

2.   **What is the management of this patient?**
     a.   Peritoneal dialysis
     b.   50–75% fluid restriction
     c.   IV 0.9% NaCl + 5% glucose (maintenance plus 7% deficit over 48 h)
     d.   Referral to nephrologist
     e.   None of the above

Case 15

A 2-month-old baby girl presents with vomiting, failure to thrive, diarrhoea, jaundice, and large liver and cataract.

Na	136 mmol/l
K	4 mmol/l
U	3.8 mm/h
Cr	60 mmol/l
LFT and clotting	Normal except high bilirubin 230 mmol/l (95% conjugated)

Urine:

Reducing substances	+++
RBC	0
Glucose	0

1. **What is the most likely diagnosis?**
    a. Septicaemia
    b. Liver failure
    c. Galactosaemia
    d. Viral hepatitis
    e. None of the above

2. **What one test will confirm the diagnosis?**
    a. Liver biopsy
    b. RBC assay of galactose-1-phosphate uridyltransferase
    c. Cranial MRI scan
    d. Urine toxicology
    e. White cell enzymes

Case 16

A 6-year-old presents with jaundice, lethargy and not feeling well.

AP	1200
Albumin	60
ALT	200
APTT	90 s
Bili	200
INR	1.3
Caeruloplasmin	11 mg/dl (>20 mg/dl)
Urinary copper	200 μg (<100 μg)

1. **What is the most likely diagnosis?**

2. **What other two tests may help to confirm the diagnosis?**

3. **What are the three steps of management?**

Case 17

A 5-year-old boy presents with a history of nose bleeding and easy bruising.

BT   9 min
APTT 70 s
PT   60 s
Plt $250 \times 10^9/l$
FVII Low
TT   10 s

1. **What is the likely diagnosis?**
   a. Haemophilia A
   b. Von Willebrand disease
   c. Christmas disease
   d. Vitamin K deficiency
   e. Factor VII deficiency

2. **What other two tests will help in diagnosis?**
   a. Ristocetin-induced platelet aggregation
   b. vWF
   c. Factor IX
   d. Fibrinogen level
   e. Factor VII

Case 18

An 8-month-old infant presents with seizures and lethargy.

Na	136 mmol/l
K	4.6 mmol/l
U	2.8 mm/h
Cr	50 mmol
AP	800 mmol/l
ALT	30 mmol/l
Bili	9 mmol/l
Ca	1.61 mmol/l (corrected 1.71 mmol/l)
25(OH)D	12 nmol/l (20 nmol/l)

1. **What is the diagnosis?**

2. **What two further tests may help in diagnosis?**

3. **What is the treatment?**

Case 19

A 13-year-old girl who has been a vegetarian for the last 3 years complains of lethargy, abdominal pain and occasional excessive periods.

Hb	8.6 g/dl
WCC	$6.1 \times 10^9/l$ (N 1.2, L 5)
Plt	$80 \times 10^9/l$
MCHC	95 g/l
MCV	75 fl

Increased segmentation of polymorphonuclear leukocytes on blood film

1. **What are the most likely diagnoses?**
   a. Folic acid deficiency
   b. Vitamin B_{12} deficiency
   c. Vitamin B_6 deficiency
   d. Vitamin B_1 deficiency
   e. None of the above

2. **What further two tests would confirm the diagnoses?**
   a. Jejunal biopsy
   b. Plasma vitamin B_{12} level
   c. Folic acid level
   d. Vitamin B_1 level
   e. Vitamin B_6 level

Case 20

A 5-year-old boy is referred with a history of nocturnal enuresis that had caused concern for the last 3 months. Recently, he has started to suffer daytime enuresis and faecal soiling. On examination, decreased ankle jerks and a reduction in sensitivity over the saddle area are noted. Spinal X-ray is normal and there is no birthmark on his back.

1. At which spine level is the lesion?

2. List three important causes.

3. Name one single investigation of value in this case.

Case 11

1. Acute glomerulonephritis
2. Blood pressure
   Daily weight

Acute glomerulonephritis

Glomerular lesions in acute glomerulonephritis (AGN) are the result of glomerular deposition or in situ formation of immune complexes. Histopathological changes include swelling of the glomerular tufts and infiltration with polymorphonucleocytes. Immunofluorescence reveals deposition of immunoglobulins and complement.

The presentation is classically with oedema, frequently including the face, specifically the periorbital area. There is hypertension in as many as 80% of patients in all populations affected. Gross haematuria and hypocomplementaemia is another feature of AGN.

Management includes restricting fluid to up to one third of daily requirements, and giving phenoxymethylpenicillin. If blood pressure is high, consider labetalol and/or furosemide. Discuss with the nephrologist and transfer if the patient goes into renal failure, or severe hypertension may lead to encephalopathy.

In severe hypertension, with or without end-organ insufficiency, the agents useful in treating hypertension include calcium channel blockers and nitroprusside. Note that beta-blocking agents or angiotensin-converting enzyme (ACE) inhibitors may not be useful unless administered with vasodilators and diuretics, because plasma renin activity levels are reduced. In most patients with less severe hypertension, captopril should decrease blood pressure in less than 1 hour. Note that, since renin activity is depressed, use of captopril carries the risk of hyperkalaemia. Monitor serum potassium closely.

In post-streptococcal nephritis, the long-term prognosis is good and >98% of individuals are asymptomatic after 5 years. From 1% to 3% of all patients with AGN may develop chronic renal failure.

Case 12

1. Reye syndrome
2. Clotting screen
   Liver biopsy

Reye syndrome

Reye syndrome (RS) is a rare illness that can affect the blood, liver and brain of someone who has recently had a viral infection.

Symptoms include nausea and vomiting; listlessness; personality change such as irritability, combativeness or confusion; delirium; convulsions; and loss of consciousness. It can lead to coma and brain death. It primarily affects children, but can also affect adults. The cause remains unknown. Taking aspirin increases the risk in children under the age of 12 years. RS is often misdiagnosed as encephalitis, meningitis, diabetes, drug overdose, poisoning, sudden infant death syndrome or psychiatric illness.

There is no cure for RS, and supportive treatment only is needed during the acute phase.

Case 13

1. DKA
2. IV 0.9% NaCl (240 ml)
   IV insulin
   IV 0.45% NaCl and 5% glucose (3750 ml over 48 hours)
   KCl 20 mmol for each litre of IV fluid

Diabetic ketoacidosis

Ketoacidosis can be defined as a triad of hyperglycaemia, ketonaemia and acidaemia. The diagnostic criteria include:

- Blood glucose >13.9 mmol/L or 250 mg/dl
- pH <7.3
- Serum bicarbonate <15 mEq/L
- Urinary ketones >+++
- Serum osmolality variable.

If the patient is comatose, it is very important to obtain a history about the duration of symptoms. If the patient is known to have diabetes, note when the last insulin was given. DKA occurs most commonly with type 1 diabetes but can also occur with type 2 diabetes. The commonest precipitating factors for DKA in a known diabetic patient are infection, not taking insulin, or any other medical illness. It may be the first presentation of diabetes mellitus.

The main goals of treating a patient presenting with DKA are improving circulatory volume and tissue perfusion, reducing blood glucose and serum osmolality towards normal levels, clearing ketones from serum and urine at a steady rate, correcting electrolyte imbalances, and identifying precipitating factors.

The restoration of extracellular fluid volume through the intravenous administration of a physiological saline (0.9% NaCl) solution is the first step in treating DKA. By initiating this, the intravascular volume will be restored, other hormones decreased and the blood glucose level lowered. As a result of all of these, insulin sensitivity may be augmented.

Insulin infusion should be started according to the protocol, aiming to lower the blood glucose by 3–4 mmol/l per hour. When blood glucose falls to <12 mmol/l, then shift fluid to 0.45% NaCl and 5% glucose. As soon as insulin is started, add KCl 20 mmol for every litre of IV fluid; aiming to correct the dehydration over 48 hours, and usually the patient's deficit between 7% and 10%. Total fluid can be calculated as deficit = (weight × 10 × % deficit) + maintenance over 48 hours. Bicarbonate supplement is no longer used. Cerebral oedema is one of the complications that may occur with DKA treatment, especially if fluid is given too fast and glucose lowered too fast as well.

Case 14

1. SIADH
2. 50–70% fluid restriction

Syndrome of inappropriate ADH secretion

Antidiuretic hormone (ADH) is secreted by the posterior pituitary gland (neurohypophysis), and acts on the kidneys to induce water retention primarily at the level of the collecting ducts. The syndrome of inappropriate ADH secretion (SIADH) results from *inappropriate* ADH secretion resulting in inappropriate retention of ingested/infused water. It is important to note that although water excretion is impaired, *salt handling is NORMAL*.

Patients may present with headache, vomiting, hyponatraemia, nausea, decreased reflexes, lethargy or restlessness. Seizures, coma and death may occur if the condition is not recognized early and treated adequately.

SIADH may be caused by infection (CNS, lungs), stroke, trauma, leukaemia, lymphoma, neuroblastoma, CNS tumours, and drugs (carbamazepine, NSAIDs, SSRIs, cyclophosphamide and vincristine). Major surgery, AIDS and pulmonary diseases also cause SIADH. The diagnosis can be made from biochemical results, which include hyponatraemia, serum osmolality < 280 mosmol/l, urine Na > 20 mmol/l and urine osmolality > serum osmolality. Finding the cause and treating it is the priority. Fluid restriction up to one third of daily maintenance is the initial therapy.

Case 15

1. Galactosaemia
2. RBC assay of galactose-1-phosphate uridyltransferase

Galactosaemia

Galactosaemia is an autosomal recessive disorder characterized by elevated concentrations of galactose in the blood resulting from the absence or dysfunction of any of the three enzymes responsible for the transformation of galactose to glucose, i.e. D-galactose-1-phosphotransferase, α-D-galactose-1-phosphate uridyltransferase or UDP-glucose-4-epimerase.

The gene for galactosaemia has been identified in some patients. Mutations in the *GALE*, *GALK1* and *GALT* genes cause galactosaemia. Symptoms associated with galactosaemia in the newborn period can include vomiting, diarrhoea, dehydration, jaundice, hepatic failure, hypoglycaemia, cataracts and developmental retardation. Galactosaemia may be suspected if sepsis is due to *Escherichia coli*. If left untreated, galactosaemia may result in cirrhosis of the liver, mental retardation, cataract formation, and kidney damage. Treatment consists of removal of galactose and its major derivative from the food of the newborn. This must be maintained through life.

Screening for galactosaemia

The Gal-1-PUT (galactose-1-phosphate uridyltransferase) assay should be abnormal in all severely galactosaemic infants even if the specimen is obtained before lactose is ingested. If the newborn has had an exchange transfusion, this will be very difficult to measure. If some babies are fed soya milk, the blood glucose will be normal. If the urine shows non-glucose-reducing substances then galactosaemia should be considered as a diagnosis.

Case 16

1. Wilson disease
2. Liver biopsy
   Slit-lamp eye examination
3. Low-copper diet
   Penicillamine
   Liver transplant

Wilson disease

Wilson disease is inherited as an autosomal recessive disorder of copper metabolism. It is characterized by excessive deposition of copper in the kidney, liver, brain and other tissues. The genetic defect has been localized to chromosome arm 13q. Patients with Wilson disease usually present with liver disease during the first decade of life or with neuropsychiatric illness during the third decade. The diagnosis is confirmed by measurement of serum caeruloplasmin, urinary copper excretion and hepatic copper content, as well as the detection of Kayser–Fleischer rings.

Treatment includes the use of chelating agents, e.g. penicillamine. Zinc and pyridoxine can also help. Orthotopic liver transplantation can be a curative treatment option for Wilson disease. Symptomatic treatment for portal hypertension, renal failure and eye problems is essential until liver transplant is achieved.

Case 17

1. Factor VII deficiency
2. Factor IX
   Factor VII

Factor VII deficiency

This inherited autosomal recessive disorder is very rare. Bleeding does not necessarily correlate with the level of factor VII in the blood. Factor VII is vitamin K-dependent and usually formed in the liver with only 1% in the active form. Factor VII deficiency can present as early as the first 6 months of life with either fatal GIT or CNS bleeding. The commonest presentation is epistaxis or other mucosal bleeding. Haemarthrosis is another presentation with frequent bruising. The prothrombin time (PT) is prolonged and the International Normalized Ratio (INR) is elevated. The activated thromboplastin time (APTT) is normal. Fresh frozen plasma (FFP) is best to replace factor VII deficiency. Recombinant activated factor VII (rFVIIa) was originally developed to treat patients with haemophilia and inhibitors, but it can be used at lower doses for patients with congenital FVII deficiency.

Case 18

1. Rickets
2. X-ray of wrists and elbow
   Vitamin D level
3. Calcium supplement
   Vitamin D
   Referral to dietician

Nutritional rickets

Rickets usually occurs when the metabolites of vitamin D are deficient in the food. Infants and children who are breast-fed are more at risk than others, as are children with dark skin who do not have enough exposure to the sun, especially in the northern hemisphere.

Cholecalciferol (vitamin D_3) is formed in the skin from 5-dihydrotachysterol. Vitamin D_3 or vitamin D_2 may be ingested as fish liver oil or irradiated ergosterol from plant sources. After this, hydroxylation occurs in two steps. Step one occurs at position 25 in the liver, producing calcidiol (25-hydroxycholecalciferol), which is the circulating reserve compound, while step 2 occurs in the kidney at position 1, where it undergoes hydroxylation to the active metabolite calcitriol (1,25-dihydroxycholecalciferol), which acts as a hormone.

Calcitriol has effects on three sites in the body:

- It promotes absorption of calcium and phosphorus from the intestine.
- It increases reabsorption of phosphate in the kidney.

- It acts on bone to release calcium and phosphate.
- It may also directly facilitate calcification.

These can increase the concentrations of calcium and phosphate in extra-cellular fluid. This can lead to the calcification of osteoid, primarily at the metaphyseal growing ends of bones but also throughout all osteoid in the skeleton. Parathyroid hormone facilitates the 1-hydroxylation step in vitamin D metabolism and, along with calcitrol and calcitonin, plays a role in calcium regulation. If the calcitriol levels become very low, hypocalcaemia develops, which stimulates parathyroid hormone, which in turn increases renal phosphate loss, which can lead to further reduction in calcification.

Severe intestinal malabsorption and diseases of the liver or kidney may produce the clinical and secondary biochemical picture of nutritional rickets. The anticonvulsant drugs phenobarbital and phenytoin accelerate metabolism of calcidiol, which may lead to insufficiency and rickets, particularly in children who are kept indoors in institutions.

Case 19

1. Vitamin B_{12} or folic acid deficiency
2. Vitamin B_{12} and folic acid levels

Macrocytic anaemia

In macrocytic anaemia, the red cells are larger and the MCV is greater than 100 fl (normal <90 fl).

Causes

Macrocytic anaemia may be due to either vitamin B_{12} or folic acid deficiency. In vitamin B_{12} deficiency, it could be due to:

- Autoimmune causes, e.g. addisonian pernicious anaemia (80%)
- GIT surgery such as gastrectomy or ileal resection
- Bacterial overgrowth
- HIV infection
- Dietary deficiency in strict vegans
- Pernicious anaemia (rarely occurs in the newborn)

In folate deficiency, it could be due to:

- Dietary deficiency (commonest cause)
- Malabsorption due to various causes
- Increased demands, including haemolysis and leukaemia and rapid cell turnover, as may occur in some skin diseases
- Increased urinary excretion, which may occur in heart failure, acute hepatitis and haemolysis
- Drug-induced deficiency (alcohol, anticonvulsants, methotrexate, sulfasalazine and trimethoprim – but the last only if in high dose and for a prolonged course)

Causes of non-megaloblastic anaemia in children include:

- Liver disease
- Severe hypothyroidosis
- Reticulocytosis
- Other blood disorders, including aplastic anaemia, red-cell aplasia, and myeloid leukaemia
- Drugs that affect DNA synthesis, such as azathioprine

Case 20

1. S1–S4
2. Spinal space-occupying lesion (neuroblastoma, sarcoma)
   Spinal dysraphism
   Trauma
3. MRI of spine with contrast

Differential diagnosis of spinal cord injuries

Lesion	Signs
Lesion at level C1–C2	Complete quadriplegia, respiratory paralysis
Lesion at level C5–C6	Quadriplegia, preservation of diaphragmatic movement, sensory level at upper thoracic level with preservation of sensation over lateral aspects of the arm
Lesion at level T12–L1	Paraplegia, sensory level at inguinal folds, loss of sphincter control
Brown-Séquard syndrome *Unilateral lesions*	Unilateral paralysis ipsilateral to affected side, unilateral disturbances of deep sensation, disturbances of position and vibration sense ipsilateral to paralysis Unilateral (contralateral to lesion) disturbances of superficial (pain and thermal) sensation
Spinal hemiplegia *Unilateral lesions*	Either purely motor, respecting the face, or associated with sensory deficits
Central cord lesions	Upper limbs affected > lower limbs, lower motor neurone involvement of upper limbs, disturbances in pain and thermal sensation below the level of the lesion
Anterior spinal syndrome	Paraplegia, loss of pain and thermal sensation, preservation of deep sensation, may be due to anterior spinal artery compression

Spinal MRI and nerve conduction study are the most reliable diagnostic tests, but a very thorough neurological examination is still the easiest and simplest way to make a diagnosis.

Case 21

A 4-month-old infant presents with a history of failure to thrive. His liver is 4–5 cm enlarged and he has cardiomegaly. Examination reveals a gallop rhythm and engorgement of pedal veins. Investigations show:

CXR	Haziness of both hilar zones, extending to both lower and upper lobes of lungs
WCC	10×10^9/l
Hb	4.9 g/dl
Plt	300×10^9/l
MCV	93 fl
Coombs test	Negative
U	4 mmol/l
Cr	35 µmol/l
Bone marrow	Normal cellularity, reduced normoblasts

1. What is the diagnosis?

2. What is the most likely underlying cause?

3. What is the inheritance of this disease?

Case 22

A 9-year-old boy is referred with an intermittent history of haematuria and progressive hearing loss. His urinary investigations reveal:

RBC	++++
Proteinuria	+
Creatinine clearance	Normal

1. What is the most likely diagnosis?

2. What is the inheritance of this condition?

3. What is the prognosis for any affected female sibling?

Case 23

A 3-year-old boy has a history of failure to thrive. There is no diarrhoea or vomiting. His mother says that he does get warm from time to time. She changes his nappy up to 12 times per day. He wakes up crying, asking for a drink.

Na	147 mmol/l
K	3.6 mmol/l
U	2.5 mmol/l
Cr	48 µmol/l
Ca	2.56 mmol/l
PO$_4$	1.84 mmol/l
Alb	47 g/l
ALP	278 IU/l
Serum osmolality	292 mmol/kg
Urine amino acid	Normal
Renal US	Normal
MRI of head	Normal
Serum amino acid	Normal
Urine pH	5.0

1. What is the likely diagnosis?

2. Which other two tests would you do?

3. How will you investigate further?

Case 24

A 10-year-old girl presents with a UTI and abdominal pain. She is known to suffer from myopia. She has been tested in the past, and her blood has shown a high level of methionine. Skin biopsy with a fibroblast culture shows a cystathionine β-synthase deficiency. Her sister died aged 25 years with a clotting disorder.

Urine analysis:

Protein	+
WCC	15 leukocytes/mm^3
Organisms	–ve

1. What is the most likely diagnosis?

2. What other test will aid diagnosis?

3. List the other features or signs of this underlying condition

Case 25

A 2-day-old preterm baby presents with persistent bile-stained vomiting 16 hours post delivery. His birth weight was 2.4 kg, and his weight had fallen further, down to 2.00 kg. Investigations revealed:

Plasma
Na	120 mmol/l
K	3.0 mmol/l
HCO^{-3}	35 mmol/l
U	26 µmol/l

Urine:
Na	10 mmol/l
K	39 mmol/l
U	280 mmol/l

1. List three abnormalities identified by these investigations.

2. What is the most likely diagnosis?

3. What are the three most likely causes?

Case 26

A 22-month-old boy presents with a history of progressive loss of vision. He initially presented to his GP at 17 months of age because of concerns that he was not able to follow objects. His mother was reassured. He was admitted for further investigations 3 weeks later. A CT scan was performed. It revealed a large suprasellar lesion containing areas of calcification.

1. What other clinical tests are indicated?

2. What is the most likely diagnosis?

3. List three investigations of benefit.

Case 27

A 6-year-old girl presents with purpura. She has shotty palpable occipital and left cervical lymph nodes. Examination of her limbs reveals an absent right thumb. She suffers with mild mental retardation.

1. What is the diagnosis?

2. What other physical signs would you look for?

3. What investigations are indicated?

Case 28

A 10-year-old boy presents with a history of generalized pain, high fever and aches for the last 2 days. Both liver and spleen are palpable, measuring 3 cm.

He lives near a lake and has been swimming in this lake from time to time during the summer holiday. He is from the Middle East. The following results were obtained:

Hb	11.5 g/dl
WCC	3.2×10^9/l (N 40%, polymorphonuclear leukocytes 70%)
Plt	200×10^9/l
Na	133 mmol/l
K	3.5 mmol/l
U	7.5 mmol/l
Cr	80 µmol/l
CSF:	
Glucose	4.1 mmol/l
No organisms	
Protein	30 mg/l

1. What is the most likely diagnosis?

2. Give one test to confirm your diagnosis.

Case 29

A newborn baby started to fit at the age of 3 hours. The mother required IV fluids of 5% glucose for 12 hours up to 150 ml/kg.

Glc	3.4 mmol/l
Blood, urine, and CSF cultures after 48 hours with no growth	
Ca	2.21 mmol/l
Mg	0.90 mmol/l
PO$_4$	1.21 mmol/l
Hb	17.3 g/dl
WCC	6.7×10^9/l
Plt	195×10^9/l
Urine:	
WCC	1
RBC	0 epithelial cast + Gram stain
CSF:	
WCC	7
RBC	10
Protein	0.34 g
Glucose	2.1 mmol/l
No organism	

1. What is the most likely cause of the fits?

2. How can they be prevented?

Case 30

A 2-day-old infant had apnoea attacks and floppiness, and needed ventilation for 17 days. Since he has been off the ventilator, he has frequently had the hiccups.

Plasma AA	Normal, apart from elevated glycerol at 597 µmol/l (100–330)
Plasma NH_4	80 µmol/l (<200)
Plasma lactate	2.1 mmol/l (2–4)
Plasma electrolytes and urea	Normal, no ketonuria
CSF lactate	2.1 mmol/l
CSF/plasma ratio for glycerol	0.35

1. What is the diagnosis?
2. What other investigations will you ask for?

Case 21

1. Congestive heart failure
2. Diamond–Blackfan anaemia
3. Autosomal recessive

Pure red cell aplasia

This is characterized by normochromic, normocytic anaemia, reticulocytopenia, normal cellular bone marrow with selective red cell precursor reduction, normal or low white cell count, and normal or high platelet count. The inheritance is unknown.

About 95% of cases occur before 2 years of age; sometimes the condition can occur up to the age of 6 years. The early introduction of steroids is said to reduce the incidence of resistance to therapy. Steroids are usually started with a high dose for 2 weeks, which is then reduced to a very low dose on alternate days. Attempts to stop alternate steroid therapy usually end in success. If there is no response to steroids, regular transfusion with chelation for 6 days per week is required.

Other causes of pure red cell aplasia

- Thymoma
- Lymphoid malignancy
- Systemic lupus erythematosus
- Juvenile chronic arthritis
- Viruses: B19 parvovirus, EBV, hepatitis A, B, C, HIV
- Idiopathic
- Pregnancy
- Drugs: anticonvulsants (e.g. carbamazepine, sodium valproate), antibiotics (chloramphenicol, sulphonamides and isoniazid), azathioprine

Case 22

1. Alport syndrome
2. X-linked dominant
3. Good

Causes of haematuria

Interstitial	Vascular	Urinary tract	Immune	Basement membrane
Pyelonephritis	Trauma	Bacterial infection	Acute glomerulonephritis	Alport syndrome
Renal tuberculosis	Sickle cell disease/trait	Cystitis (viral or chemical)	Henoch–Schönlein purpura	Benign familial haematuria
Nephrocalcinosis	Renal vein thrombosis	Urethritis	IgA glomerulonephritis	Nail–patella syndrome
Metabolic (Fabry disease)	Renal artery Thrombosis	Obstruction or reflux	SLE	Diabetic nephropathy
Interstitial nephritis	Arteriovenous malformation	Tumour	Mesangioproliferative glomerulonephritis	
Nephrotoxins (analgesics)	Malignant Hypertension	Hypercalciuria	Minimal change glomerulonephritis	
Cystic renal disease	Congestive heart failure	Nephrolithiasis	Membranoproliferative glomerulonephritis	
Hydronephrosis	Coagulopathy		Systemic vasculitis	
Tumours	Thrombocytopenia		Amyloidosis	
Acute tubular necrosis			Shunt nephritis	
			Goodpasture disease	
			HUS	

Alport syndrome

Presentation

Patients with Alport syndrome mostly present with asymptomatic macroscopic haematuria. Another presentation is with progressive sensorineural hearing loss; 10% have associated eye problems (cataract, macular lesions).

Inheritance

Alport syndrome is inherited as an X-linked dominant, autosomal dominant trait or autosomal recessive; 20% of patients have no family history. It is more severe in males than females. Males develop end-stage renal failure in the second or third decade of life.

Prognosis and management

Females always have normal kidney function but have sensorineural hearing loss and a normal lifespan. Dialysis and kidney transplant is the mode of treatment in males. If renal biopsy is done early, it will show only slight changes. Later on, it shows mesangial proliferation and capillary wall thickening, which will lead to progressive glomerular sclerosis, total atrophy and fibrosis. All immunological studies are negative.

If the family history of haematuria is negative and there is only intermittent haematuria, the patient needs reassurance and follow-up after a year. If the patient remains asymptomatic then he/she can be discharged from the clinic, but if there is anxiety and persistent haematuria, renal biopsy should be performed as above.

Case 23

1. Diabetes insipidus (DI)
2. Cranial CT scan or MRI
   Baseline hormonal assay (GH, midnight and morning cortisol and TSH, T$_4$)
3. Water deprivation test

Main characteristic features of diabetes insipidus

	Central DI	Nephrogenic DI
Inheritance	Sporadic	X-linked recessive
Aetiology	Failure of ADH production: Idiopathic (familial) Post-traumatic CNS neoplasia Post-hypophysectomy Infections (encephalitis, meningitis) Vascular (aneurysm/ thrombosis)	Tubules unresponsive to ADH: Obstructive uropathy Potassium depletion Hypercalcaemia Sickle cell anaemia Chronic renal failure Drugs (amphotericin, tetracycline)
Polyuria	Prominent	Mild
Polydipsia	Yes	Yes
Glycosuria	No	No
Fasting plasma osmolality	>95 mmol/kg	>290 mmol/kg
Urine osmolality with desmopressin	>800 mmol/kg	<200–300 mmol/kg
Plasma Na	High	High
ADH level	Undetectable	High
Treatment	Desmopressin (intranasal, oral, IM)	Indometacin, chlorothiazide, diet low in sodium and protein

Case 24

1. Homocystinuria
2. Nitroprusside test
3. Cardiovascular system, CNS and eyes

	Homocystinuria	Marfan syndrome
Inheritance	Autosomal recessive	Autosomal dominant
Enzyme defect	Cystathionine synthetase (type I)	None
	Methylcobalamin formation (type II)	
	Methylenetetrahydrofolate reductase (type III)	
Ocular	Lens subluxation (up)	Lens subluxation (down)
Skeletal	Tall, thin and long limbs	Same as homocystinuria
	Scoliosis	
	Pectus excavatum	
	Crowded teeth	
	Osteoporosis	
Heart defect	None	Aortic valve regurgitation
		Mitral valve prolapse
Embolic phenomena	Present	None
Intelligence	50% normal	40–50% normal
Complication	Optic atrophy	
	Cor pulmonale	
	Severe hypertension	
Diagnosis	Increase in urine excretion of methionine and homocystine	Normal plasma and urine
	Low plasma cystine	amino acids
	Liver biopsy and cultured fibroblasts for enzymatic assay	Clinical
Treatment	High dose of vitamin B_6 (I)	Valvoplasty
	Vitamin B_{12} (II)	Lens replacement
	Vitamin B_6, B_{12}, folic acid and methionine supplement (III)	

Case 25

1. Na low
    K low in plasma, high in urine
    High urinary/plasma urea ratio
2. Pre-renal failure secondary to GIT obstruction
3. Peripheral vasodilatation, e.g. sepsis
    Hypovolaemia, e.g. diarrhoea, GIT obstruction
    Cardiac failure

Acute pre-renal failure

Causes

Pre-renal	Renal	Post-renal
Hypovolaemia, e.g. DKA	Hypovolaemia	Posterior urethral valves
Haemorrhage, gastroenteritis	Disease of kidney, e.g. acute glomerulonephritis	Crystals (uric acid)
Peripheral vasodilatation, e.g. sepsis	Haemolytic uraemic syndrome, cortical necrosis	Neurogenic bladder
Cardiac failure	Severe UTI	Surgical accident
Bilateral renal vessel occlusion	Nephrotoxins	Calculus
GIT obstruction	Myoglobinuria	Ureterocele
	Haemoglobinuria	Tumours
		Trauma

Diagnosis

Features of renal failure are oliguria, oedema, acidotic breathing and drowsiness. Acute hypertensive encephalopathy may occur.

	Pre-renal	Renal
Na (urine)	<20 mmol/l	>30 mmol/l
U:P osmolality ratio	>1:1.5	<1:1
U:P urea ratio	>10	<10
Urine osmolality	>400	<400
U:P creatinine ratio	>20	<20

Case 26

1. Blood pressure
    Visual fields/acuity
    Fundus examination
2. Craniopharyngioma

3. Urea and electrolytes, glucose, osmolality (urine and plasma)
   Random plasma cortisol, GH, LHRH, TSH
   Head MRI scan

Craniopharyngioma

Craniopharyngioma arises from the remnants of the embryonic Rathke's pouch. These tumours represent about 50% of midline tumours in infancy and childhood (Bailey et al 1990).

Clinical features

These include growth retardation and visual disturbances in children and failure of sexual maturation in adolescents. Bitemporal hemianopia is present in half of patients and homonymous hemianopia in 10–20%. Visual acuity is diminished in one or both eyes in every child (Hoffmann et al 1977). Unilateral loss of vision may occur rapidly, as in optic neuritis. Focal neurological signs are uncommon. A quarter of cases suffer from hydrocephalus with headache and papilloedema.

Investigations

Fifty per cent of patients have GH deficiency. Gonadotropic hormones are low in 50% of pubertal patients. TSH and ACTH deficiencies are less common in non-operated patients but appear in most cases after the operation. Hypothalamic involvement may cause diabetes insipidus or ADH deficiency with lethargy and hypotension. Lateral extension of the tumour may cause third- and fifth-nerve palsy. Calcification is a frequent and important feature of craniopharyngioma. MRI is the first choice of imaging if available.

Management

Subtotal resection followed by radiotherapy is the usual approach for treatment. Endocrine disturbances are exacerbated with the development of diabetes insipidus in 75% of patients. A variety of psychological deficits are often present. Epilepsy is present in 10–12% of patients. Patients who have not received radiotherapy have a higher IQ than those who have (Pierre-Kahn 1988).

Case 27

1. Fanconi anaemia
2. Hyperpigmented patches
   Absence of radial bone
3. Full blood count
   Chromosomal analysis

Fanconi anaemia

Fanconi anaemia (FA) is nearly always inherited as an autosomal recessive trait. There are at least 13 genes mutations of which are known to cause FA: *FANCA, B, C, D1, D2, E, F, G, I, J, L, M* and *N* (of these, *FANCB*, which is on the X chromosome, gives rise to the very rare cases of X-linked inheritance). Many patients will develop acute myeloid leukaemia. Older patients may develop malignancies of GIT, brain, neck and anus.

Patients can present with short stature and skin pigmentation (café-au-lait spots). Petechiae and bruises are the first haematological symptoms a patient may present with. Thumb and radial abnormalities may be observed in 40% of patients. Other abnormalities include abnormal male gonads (30%), microcephaly (25%), eye anomalies (20%), structural renal defects (20%), low birthweight (10%), developmental delay (10%), and abnormal ears or hearing (10%).

Case 28

1. Leptospirosis
2. Stool/blood, urine cultures
   Weil test (serology)

Leptospirosis (Weil disease)

Leptospira is transmitted to humans from infected animal urine (rats or other rodents). The organisms migrate to the capillaries and cause micro-capillary damage everywhere, leading to muscle pain, renal failure, liver failure, meningitis and rashes. There are different species of *Leptospira*, the commonest being *L. icterohaemorrhagiae* (rats), *L. canicola* (dogs) and *L. pomona* (pigs).

Clinical features

The incubation period varies from a few days to 3 weeks; the disease usually starts with the abrupt onset of fever followed by other features – lethargy, jaundice, rashes, meningism, and renal, liver and cardiac failure. There is a pancytopenia with a high lymphocyte count in the CSF and no organism. The ESR is high. The haemagglutination test is positive in the second week of illness and blood culture is positive in the first week of illness. Urine will be positive after 3 weeks of the illness. *Leptospira* is sensitive to penicillin; tetracycline for 7 days is also effective. There is a live vaccine stock for prevention for those travelling to endemic areas.

Q fever presents like leptospirosis and can be differentiated by culture. Brucellosis is also transmitted from animal to human, and can present with intermittent fever and joint pain. It can affect any organ, but most commonly the skeletal, gastrointestinal and respiratory systems. Diagnosis is by finding raised titres for *Brucella* by agglutination test. It is also sensitive to tetracycline and co-trimoxazole.

Case 29

1. Hyponatraemia secondary to hypervolaemia and oxytocin
2. Maintenance fluid to mother
   Oxytocin only during second stage

Hyponatraemia (Na <130 mmol/l)

Aetiology

Loss of sodium in excess of water	Gain of water in excess of sodium
External loss	SIADH
Gastro-intestinal – diarrhoea	Renal failure
Skin – excessive sweating	Excessive water intake
Third-space losses – burns	Oedematous states
Renal salt loss	
Renal – RTA, diuretic therapy	
Non-renal CAH/Addison disease	

Investigation of hyponatraemia

Aetiology	Loss of water in excess of Na		Gain of water in excess of sodium	
Investigation	External loss	Renal salt loss	Oedematous states	SIADH
Volume	Reduced	Increased	Reduced	Reduced
Urine Na	<20 mmol/l	>20 mmol/l	<20 mmol/l	>20 mmol/l
Urine osmolarity	>500 mmol/l	Isotonic	>500 mmol/l	Hyperosmolar
Plasma urea	Increased	Increased	Normal or increased	Normal or reduced
Plasma osmolarity	Reduced	Reduced	Reduced	Reduced

Case 30

1. Non-ketotic hyperglycinaemia
2. Brain MRI and EEG

	Ketotic hyperglycinaemia (organic acidaemias)	Non-ketotic hyperglycinaemia
Inheritance	AR	AR
Ammonia	High	Normal
Ketoacidosis	Abnormal	Normal
Glucose	Low	Normal
Lactate	High	Normal
Glycine	High	Normal
Neutrophils	Low	Normal
Thrombocytes	Low	Normal
CSF/plasma glycine	Normal	Increased ratio
Seizures	Multiple seizures	Myoclonic type
EEG	Generalized activity	Suppression-burst, hypsarrhythmia
MRI	Non-specific changes	Progressive cerebral atrophy and demyelination of supratentorial white matter

EMQs

For the following scenarios, choose the diagnosis from List A and match it with the diagnostic genetic abnormalities on molecular genetic testing from List B.

Case 31

A 4-year-old boy has a history of developmental delay, large forehead, prominent chin and long ears. He also has macro-orchidism.

Case 32

A newborn baby has dysmorphic features of microcephaly, micrognathia and down-slanting palpebral fissures. He also has a cat-like cry.

Case 33

A term baby girl was born with lymphoedema on the dorsum of hands and feet. She has redundant skin on her back.

Case 34

A term baby was born with ambiguous genitalia, no dysmorphic features. A week later she presents with lethargy and vomiting and is not well. She is treated for sepsis.

Na	131 mmol/l
K	6.3 mmol/l
U	6.8 mm/h
Cr	80 mmol
Urine:	
Na	20 mmol/l (20 mmol/l)
RBC	0

Case 35

An 18-month-old boy is not walking yet. He is not able to weight-bear and neurological examination is entirely normal.

Na	136 mmol/l
K	4.3 mmol/l
U	2.8 mm/h
Cr	70 mmol
TSH	1.23
T$_4$	19.1
CK	2200 mmol/l
ESR	<1 mm/h

List A

a. Adrenoleukodystrophy
b. Cystic fibrosis
c. Beta-thalassaemia
d. Duchenne muscular dystrophy
e. Fragile X
f. Galactosaemia
g. Turner syndrome
h. Williams syndrome
i. Down syndrome
j. Marfan syndrome
k. Cri-du-chat syndrome
l. Tuberous sclerosis
m. Werdnig–Hoffmann syndrome
n. Dermatomyositis
o. Myotonic dystrophy
p. Noonan syndrome
q. Congenital adrenal hyperplasia

List B

a. Xp21
b. 6p21
c. Xq27
d. 7q31
e. Xq27
f. 45XO
g. 9q33
h. 5q
i. 5p-
j. 12q24
k. 9q13
l. 11p15
m. 9p13

EMQs

For the following data and scenarios, choose the most appropriate diagnosis from List A, the most appropriate investigations from List B and the most appropriate treatments from List C.

Case 36

A 13-year-old girl presents with tiredness, lethargy and inability to move her legs. She has been well over the last few weeks, but since the beginning of the week she has felt weak. She has never been abroad, and, apart from a mild cold 4 weeks ago, she is a healthy young girl. Lower limb reflexes are absent.

Hb	12.1 g/dl
WCC	8.9×10^9/l
N	5.3 (L 2.7, E 0.4, M 0.5, B 0.0)
Plt	310×10^9/l
Blood film	Mild neutrophilia
CRP	<5 mg/l (0–8)
Total bilirubin	11µmol/l (0–23)
ALP	170 u/l (109–272)
ALT	18 u/l (0–45)
Albumin	40 g/l (35–50)
IgG	13.2 g/l (4.9–16.1)
IgA	1.4 g/l (0.4–2)
IgM	1.2 g/l (0.05–0.2)
ESR	3 mm/h (0–10)
CSF protein	55 g/l (<20)
CSF cells	–ve
MRI	Brain and spine normal in appearance

Case 37

A 5-day-old baby presents with excessive crying, feeding less and jaundice. He is the first child to a first-cousin couple. There are no other concerns.

Hb	16 g/dl
WCC	7.9×10^9/l
N	4.3 (L 3.7, E 0.4, M 0.5, B 0.0)
Plt	191×10^9/l
PCV	60
CRP	<5 mg/l (0–8)
Total bilirubin	355 µmol/l (0–23)
Albumin	42 g/l (35-50)
ALP	190 u/l (109–272)
ALT	14 u/l (0–45
Blood culture after 48 hours	No growth
Urine	No cells and no organisms; culture shows no growth
DCT	–ve

Case 38

A 6-year-old boy presents with a temperature of 38.5 °C over the last 5 weeks. Every three days his temperature has gone up to 39.5 °C, settled after 4 days and then started again. He has been to Kenya and this temperature developed on the third day after his arrival. No one else in his family has similar problems.

Blood culture after 48 hours   No growth
Blood film on three occasions shows no parasite
Mantoux test was >15 mm
Chest X-ray reported as normal

LP	Protein	60 (<40)
	Cells	1600 (mainly lymphocytes)
	Glucose	2.1 mmol/l (blood 5.3 mmol/l)
	Gram stain	No organism
Hb		11 g/dl
WCC		8.9 × 10⁹/l
N		5.3 (L 3.7, E 0.4, M 0.5, B 0.0)
Plt		450 × 10⁹/l
CRP		25 mg/l (0–8)
Total bilirubin		15 µmol/l (0–23)
ALT		18 u/l (0–45)
ALP		2300 u/l (109–272)
Albumin		35 g/l (35–50)

Case 39

A 2-month-old girl presents with cough and not feeding well. She was full term with no previous problems. She requires 2 litres of oxygen per nasal canula and is still having episodes of coughing lasting up to 2–3 minutes. She has an apnoeic episode with one coughing episode.

CXR	Hyperinflated lungs
Blood gas:	
pH	7.32
BE	–2
P_{CO_2}	5.1 kPa
P_{O_2}	9.1 kPa
Hb	14 g/dl
WCC	11.9 × 10⁹/l
N	4.3 (L 7.7, E 0.4, M 0.5, B 0.0)
Plt	250 × 10⁹/l
CRP	<5 mg/l (0–8)
Total bilirubin	15 µmol/l (0–23)
ALP	195 u/l (109–272)
ALT	19 u/l (0–45)
Albumin	38 g/l (35–50)

Case 40

A 9-month-old girl presents with history of lethargy, not feeding very well and losing weight. She was born at term and there have been no concerns about her over the last 8 months.

Hb	10 g/dl
WCC	17.9×10^9/l
N	11.3 (L 5.7, E 1.4, M 0.5, B 0.0)
Plt	350×10^9/l
CRP	190 mg/l (0–8)
ALT	16 u/l (0–45)
Total bilirubin	9 µmol/l (0–23)
ALP	135 u/l (109–272)
Albumin	44 g/l (35–50)
Blood culture shows no growth	
MSU	+ve for nitrate and 100 leukocytes
CSF	10 red cells, no white cells and no organisms; culture shows no growth

List A

a. UTI
b. Bacterial meningitis
c. Encephalitis
d. Physiological jaundice
e. Viral hepatitis
f. TB meningitis
g. Hypothyroidism
h. Bronchiolitis
i. Malaria
j. Guillain–Barré syndrome
k. Typhoid fever
l. Bacterial endocarditis
m. Whooping cough
n. Cystic fibrosis
o. Transverse myelitis

List B

a. Nerve conduction study
b. Per nasal swab
c. Nasopharyngeal aspirate
d. Sweat test
e. Urine microscopy and culture
f. Renal ultrasound
g. EMG
h. PCR for *Mycobacterium tuberculosis*
i. Malaria antigen
j. TFT
k. Split bilirubin

List C

a. Oral trimethoprim for 5 days
b. IVIG 1mg/kg/day for 2 days
c. Nasogastric feeding
d. Oral erythromycin for 5 days
e. Phototherapy
f. Exchange transfusion
g. Intravenous ceftriaxone
h. Oral rifampicin and isoniazid for 3 months
i. Oral rifampicin, isoniazid, pyrazinamide and ethambutol for 12 months
j. Neurorehabilitation
k. IV quinine for 5 days
l. Regular physiotherapy

Case 31

1. Fragile X syndrome
2. Xq27

Fragile X syndrome

Fragile X syndrome is caused by a mutation in the *FMR1* gene, located on the X chromosome. Fragile X syndrome affects males and females of all ethnic groups. It is estimated that about 1 in 4000 to 1 in 6250 males are affected with fragile X syndrome. There are approximately half as many females with fragile X syndrome as there are males. The carrier frequency in unaffected females is 1 in 100 to 1 in 600, with one study finding a carrier frequency of 1 in 250. It is one of the most common causes of mental retardation and developmental delay. Other features that may be associated with fragile X syndrome include language delays, behavioural problems, autism or autistic-like behaviour (including poor eye contact and hand-flapping), enlarged genitalia (macro-orchidism), large or prominent ears, hyperactivity, delayed motor development, and/or poor sensory skills. Prenatal diagnosis is possible by amniocentesis, chorionic villus biopsy and percutaneous umbilical blood sampling. It is recommended that it should be offered as part of genetic counselling if a parent is known to be a carrier.

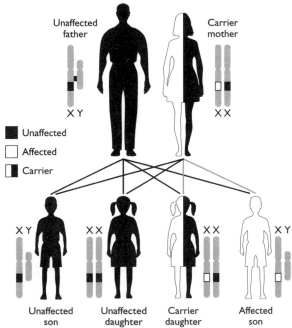

X-linked recessive, carrier mother

Unaffected father

Carrier mother

X Y

X X

■ Unaffected
□ Affected
▮ Carrier

X Y

X X

X X

X Y

Unaffected son

Unaffected daughter

Carrier daughter

Affected son

Case 32

1. Cri du chat syndrome
2. 5p–

Cri-du-chat syndrome

The syndrome is usually associated with a small head, low birthweight, poor muscle tone, microcephaly and a characteristic cry ('cat's-cry syndrome') and facial features. Some infants have language difficulties and the majority have speech delay. There is delayed walking because of poor muscle tone and the later development of scoliosis. Death occurs in infancy or early childhood.

Case 33

1. Turner syndrome
2. 45XO

Turner syndrome affects approximately 1 out of every 2500 female live births worldwide. At birth, the girls have lymphoedema affecting the dorsum of the hands and feet. Almost all patients with Turner syndrome are short. This is due to loss of the *SHOX* gene on the X chromosome, which plays a major role in long bone growth. It also explains the short fingers and increased carrying angle at the elbow joint. Most girls do not enter puberty at the normal time and may need hormonal replacement. Oestrogen can be given for breast development and other features of puberty if menses do not start by the age of 15 years. Approximately 5–10% are found to have coarctation of the aorta. Other features include bicuspid aortic valve, high blood pressure in adult life, horseshoe kidney and a high incidence of osteoporosis. Type 2 diabetes is also known to occur in patients with Turner syndrome, as is hypothyroidism. The girls have normal intelligence.

Case 34

1. Congenital adrenal hyperplasia
2. 6p21

Congenital adrenal hyperplasia

Approximately 1 in 10 000–18 000 children are born with congenital adrenal hyperplasia.

The associated features in girls include ambiguous genitalia, early appearance of pubic and armpit hair, excessive hair growth, deep voice, abnormal menstrual periods, and failure to menstruate. In boys, the features are different, but the age at which symptoms occur is similar to girls. They may present with early development of masculine characteristics, well-developed musculature, enlarged penis, small testes, and early appearance of pubic and armpit hair. Both boys and girls will be tall as children but significantly shorter than normal as adults.

Blood and urine tests in boys and girls will show:

- Abnormal salt levels in blood (serum electrolytes) and urine
- High levels of urinary 17-ketosteroids
- Normal or low urinary 17-hydroxycorticosteroids
- High levels of 17-hydroxyprogesterone
- High levels of serum DHEA sulphate
- Low levels of aldosterone and cortisol

An X-ray for bone age demonstrates markedly older bones than is normal for the child's actual age. Genetic tests can help diagnose or confirm the disease, and can be useful in the management of the condition.

Any form of cortisol (fludrocortisone and hydrocortisone) may be used in treatment, and must be taken every day. Cortisol replacement consists of hydrocortisone 12–25 mg/m²/day in two doses. The dose can be increased by 10% during infection or surgery or any stressful illness. The gender of the baby can be determined by examining the karyotype, and early reconstructive surgery should be done, especially for girls (age 2–3 months). It is necessary to monitor growth and virilization as well as 17-hydroxyprogesterone and testosterone levels. Patients also require salt and aldosterone replacement (salt, up to 5 mmol/kg/day; fludrocortisone, 100–200 µg/day in divided doses), and their blood pressure should be monitored as well as plasma renin activity and electrolytes.

Case 35

1. Duchenne muscular dystrophy
2. Xp21

Duchenne muscular dystrophy

The mean age at diagnosis of Duchenne muscular dystrophy (DMD) is 4½ years; wheelchair dependence occurs at a median age of 10 years; cardiac muscle failure develops in 15% of patients at a median age of 21½ years; smooth muscle dysfunction in the digestive or urinary tract occurs in 21% and 6% of patients, respectively, at a median age of 15 years. Death occurs at a median age of 17 years.

Pseudohypertrophy of the calves and proximal muscle weakness are the main features. Delayed walking may be the initial presentation and CK will be very high. EMG will show myopathic changes, and myofibre degeneration with fibrosis and fatty infiltration can be seen on muscle biopsy. Involvement of myocardium can start as early as 6 years of age, and there is severe cardiomyopathy by the age of 21 years. Pseudo-obstruction and gastric dilatation may occur later in life as a result of smooth muscle involvement. Walking devices, respiratory support and prevention of scoliosis are the main goals of treatment. Use of steroids can delay the need for a wheelchair, but a referral to a specialist is the best option. Genetic therapy is still in its early stages. It is aimed at restoring the reading frame in muscle cells from DMD patients through targeted modulation of dystrophin pre-mRNA splicing.

Case 36

1. Guillain–Barré syndrome
2. Nerve conduction study
3. IVIG 1 mg/kg once a day for 2 days

Guillain–Barré syndrome

Guillain–Barré syndrome (GBS) is an acquired disease of the peripheral nerves. It is characterized clinically by rapidly progressing paralysis, areflexia, variable sensory disturbance, and elevated CSF protein without pleocytosis and back pain. It affects both sexes, involves people of all ages, and is reported worldwide. It is one of the most common causes of an acute generalized paralysis.

The incidence of the disease ranges from 0.5 to 1.5 in 100 000 in individuals less than 18 years of age. Approximately 15% of children with Guillain–Barré syndrome develop respiratory failure and require mechanical ventilatory support. The prognosis for recovery in children is generally excellent, with the majority of children achieving a complete functional recovery within 6 months from the onset of illness.

Treatment of Guillain–Barré syndrome includes both important supportive measures and immunotherapies, specifically high-dose IVIG of 2 g/kg as a total dose, which can be given over either 2 days or 5 days according to local protocols.

Case 37

1. Physiological jaundice
2. Split bilirubin
3. Phototherapy

Physiological jaundice

This is the most common cause of newborn jaundice and occurs in >50% of babies. It usually disappears by 1–2 weeks of age. The levels of bilirubin are harmless and phototherapy is rarely needed unless the level is very high and the baby not fed well. If jaundice remains beyond 3 weeks of age, then a prolonged jaundice screen should be performed, including TFT, split bilirubin, LFT, urine for MSU and reducing substances, plus full general and systemic examination.

Case 38

1. TB meningitis
2. PCR from CSF for *Mycobacterium tuberculosis*

3. Oral rifampicin, isoniazid, pyrazinamide and ethambutol for 12 months.

TB meningitis

TB meningitis is always difficult to diagnose, but a good history and examination with a high index of suspicion should help in diagnosis. There are non-specific symptoms, which include headache, vomiting, photophobia and fever. Meningeal symptoms are very rare, and duration of symptoms varies from 1 to 9 months. Sudden onset of neurological deficit, ophthalmoplegia, seizure, tremor and confusion may be the presenting features. Symptom and signs of SIADH can be early features. CSF analysis and PCR for *M. tuberculosis* can be helpful, as well as CSF culture. Neuroimaging can help, as it may show meningeal enhancement or tuberculoma.

Outcome of lumbar puncture in children suspected with meningitis

A fundal examination or head CT scan prior to lumbar puncture is recommended if there is a suspicious increase in intracranial pressure. Herniation with lumbar puncture occurs in between 4.6% and 6.4% of meningitic patients.

Differential diagnosis

	Glucose (0.66% of blood level)	Protein (0.2–0.4 g/l)	Cells (newborn WCC up to 10 is normal)	Pressure (8–10 mmHg)	Culture
Bacterial meningitis	Low	High	Polymorphs	Normal or increased	Positive in many cases
Viral meningitis	Low or normal	Normal	Lymphocytes	Normal or increased	Negative (PCR helpful)
TB meningitis	Low	High (200 mg/dl)	Lymphocytes	Normal or increased	12–27% positive
Brain abscess	Low in 30%	Normal	Sterile leukocytosis	High – LP contraindicated	Sterile
Tumour	Normal or low	Normal	Sterile (malignant cells)	High – LP contraindicated	Sterile
Guillain–Barré syndrome	Normal	High	Normal	Normal	Sterile
Mycotic meningitis	Low	High	High lymphocytes	Normal	Occasional positive
Encephalitis	Normal	High	Normal or high lymphocytes	High – CT scan indicated	PCR is helpful

Treatment

The most effective antimicrobial agents in the treatment of TB meningitis include isoniazid (INH), rifampicin (RIF), pyrazinamide (PZA) and streptomycin (SM), all of which enter CSF readily in the presence of meningeal inflammation. Ethambutol is less effective in meningeal disease unless used in high doses. Children must be treated for 12 months with combination antibiotic therapy and adjunctive corticosteroids.

Case 39

1. Whooping cough
2. Per nasal swab
3. Oral erythromycin for 5 days

Whooping cough

Whooping cough is caused by infection with the bacterium *Bordetella pertussis*. Symptoms of the infection include prolonged, strong coughing spasms and vomiting because of cough and wheezing. Infants younger than 1 year are most susceptible and have the most severe symptoms, but teenagers and adults may also have similar infection and symptoms.

The first stage of whooping cough is known as the catarrhal stage, and looks like a common cold or viral URTI. It usually lasts 1–2 weeks. The second stage is called the paroxysmal stage. It is characterized by paroxysms of coughing, which may followed by a whoop. Sometimes this leads to apnoea and cyanosis and vomiting due to cough. It may last 2–6 weeks. The third stage of whooping cough is the recovery or convalescent stage. The infant recovers gradually, with the cough becoming less paroxysmal and usually disappearing over 2–3 weeks. Supportive therapy with oxygen and nutrition during the paroxysmal stage is very important. Prescribing erythromycin for 5 days is a good practice to eradicate the infection. If the infant has not been vaccinated, he or she should be given the vaccine. Parents should be shown a resuscitation video and given written information about the disease.

Case 40

1. UTI
2. Renal ultrasound
3. Intravenous ceftriaxone until sensitivities are ascertained

Urinary tract infection

There are new NICE guidelines about UTI, which many hospitals have modified. It is beyond our scope to describe them here, but they are easily available on the Internet (NICE 2007).

Questions 41–50

EMQs

For the following investigations, choose the right diagnosis from List A and the most appropriate treatments from List B.

Case 41

A 4-year-old girl presents with episodes of daydreaming.

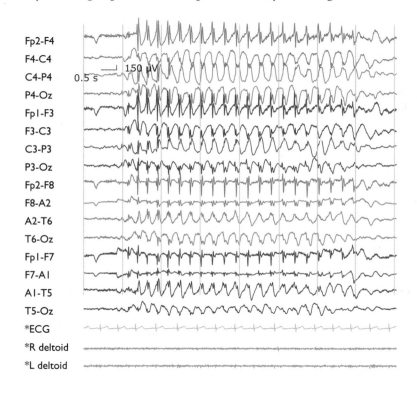

Case 42

A 4-month-old baby boy presents with a history of crying during feeding.

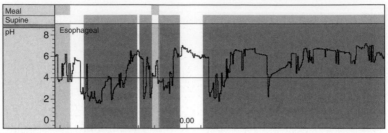

Reflux Table – ph

	Total	Upright	Supine	Meal	PostPr	PrePra
Duration of Period (min)	1d	07:10	16:49	01:20	04:04	18:35
Number of Refluxes	364	190	178	31	67	267
Number of Long Refluxes > 5 (min)	15	1	12	0	7	7
Duration of longest reflux (min)	15	5	15	3	14	15
Time pH < 4 (min)	238	72	165	13	94	131
Fraction Time pH < 4 (%)	16.5	16.8	16.4	15.8	38.4	11.8

Signature:_____

Case 43

This is an audiogram for a 3-year-old child with delayed speech:

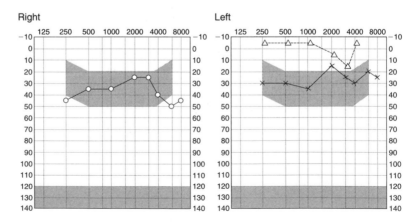

Case 44

A child presents with apnoeic spells during the night.

STUDY DURATION AND VALUES				
			PR	TIME
START DATE/TIME: 06/01/08 21:31:30	LOW SpO2:	55%	126 BPM	23:36:18
END DATE/TIME: 07/01/08 01:33:00	AVERAGE SpO2: 93%			
STUDY DURATION: 04:01:30	STD. DEV. SpO2: 6%			
			SpO2	TIME
	HIGH PR	214	98%	23:14:06
# SpO2 VALUES BELOW 85%: 208	LOW PR	99	95%	23:14:18
TOTAL DURATION BELOW 85%: 00:20:48	AVERAGE PR	142		

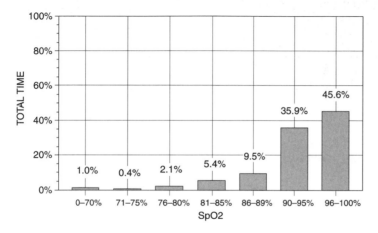

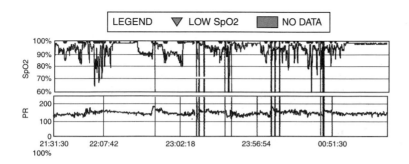

LEGEND ▼ LOW SpO2 ▨ NO DATA

Case 45

This is a recording of an ECG on a child who was resuscitated and transferred to PICU:

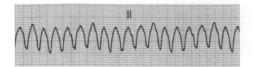

List A

a. Otitis media
b. Supraventricular tachycardia
c. Myoclonic epilepsy
d. Obstructive apnoea
e. Infantile spasms
f. Sensorineural deafness
g. Severe GOR
h. 4½ years old
i. 3 years old
j. Childhood absence epilepsy syndrome
k. Mild GOR
l. Conductive hearing loss
m. Ventricular tachycardia
n. Atrial fibrillation
o. 2½ years old
p. Moderate GOR

List B

a. Ranitidine and domperidone for 3–6 months
b. Grommet insertion
c. Cardioversion 10 J/kg
d. Urgent adenotonsillectomy
e. Levetiracetam
f. Omeprazole
g. Thick and Easy
h. Sodium valproate
i. Lamotrigine
j. Oral Augmentin for 5 days
k. IV adrenaline

EMQs

For the following scenarios, choose the most appropriate diagnosis from List A and the two most appropriate investigations from List B.

Case 46

An 18-month-old presents with a history of lethargy, losing weight and distended abdomen. There is a mass on the right side of the abdomen, which the examiner can go above and which crosses the midline. The blood pressure is 110/70 mmHg.

Hb	6.2 g/dl
WCC	9.9 × 10⁹/l
N	4.3 (L 3.7, E 1.4, M 0.5, B 0.0)
Plt	250 × 10⁹/l
CRP	35 mg/l (0–8)
Total bilirubin	11 µmol/l (0–23)
ALP	160 u/l (109–272)
ALT	19 u/l (0–45)

Abdominal ultrasound shows a right abdominal mass with calcification; no kidney tissue can be seen on the right.

Case 47

A 14-year-old boy presents with a petechial rash, bruising very easily and tiredness.

Hb	12.2 g/dl
WCC	12.9 × 10⁹/l
N	7.3 (L 5.7, E 1.4, M 0.5, B 0.0)
Plt	22 × 10⁹/l
CRP	<5 mg/l (0–8)
Total bilirubin	19 µmol/l (0–23)
ALP	370 u/l (109–272)
ALT	21 u/l (0–45)

Abdominal CT shows a large spleen, 17 cm in total, liver within normal range and paraortic large lymph nodes.

Case 48

An 11-month-old girl presents with a history of failure to thrive. She is pale, with no organomegaly and no lymphadenopathy. Her parents are from Pakistan and have been living in the UK for the last 15 years.

Hb	4.2 g/dl
WCC	15 × 10⁹/l
N	9.3 (L 6.7, E 1.4, M 0.5, B 0.0)
Plt	450 × 10⁹/l
MCV	66
Hct	<1
CRP	<5 mg/l (0–8)
Total bilirubin	7 µmol/l (0–23)
ALP	560 u/l (109–272)
ALT	14 u/l (0–45)
MCHC	77
Albumin	38 g/l (35–50)
U	2.3 mmo/l
Cr	46 mmol/l
Na	137 mmol/l
K	4.2 mmol/l
Ca	1.5 mmol/l
Corrected Ca	1.7 mmol/l
Mg	0.9 mmol/l
P	2.5 mmol/l

Case 49

A 4-year-old presents with a history of abdominal pain, pallor, jaundice and lethargy. He has been travelling with his parents over the last 2 months in South America. He first felt unwell 2 days ago.

Hb	7.2 g/dl
WCC	11 × 10⁹/l
N	7.3 (L 4.7, E 1.4, M 0.5, B 0.0)
Plt	190 × 10⁹/l
MCV	76
Hct	>3
CRP	<5 mg/l (0–8)
Total bilirubin	9 µmol/l (0–23)
ALP	240 u/l (109–272)
ALT	17 u/l (0–45)
MCHC	91
Na	139 mmol/l
Albumin	39 g/l (35–50)

Limited blood film shows target cells, Howell–Jolly bodies, abnormally shaped red cells, and anisocytosis with normochromic, normocytic anaemia.

Case 50

A 7-month-old baby boy presents to A&E with jaundice. He is pale and lethargic. Over the previous month, he has been started on solids and last week was started on malaria prophylaxis as he is travelling with his parents to Kenya this week.

Hb	8.5 g/dl
WCC	11 × 10⁹/l
N	9.3 (L 2.7, E 1.4, M 0.5, B 0.0)
Plt	210 × 10⁹/l
MCV	72
Hct	<1
CRP	<5 mg/l (0–8)
Total bilirubin	190 µmol/l (0–23)
Conjugated bilirubin	<9 mmol/l
ALP	275 u/l (109–272)
ALT	16 u/l (0–45)
MCHC	88

Blood film shows anisocytosis, polychromasia, and normochromic, normocytic anaemia.

List A

a. Elliptocytosis
b. Hepatitis
c. Sickle cell anaemia
d. Lymphoma
e. Hypocalcaemia
f. Myelodysplastic leukaemia
g. Wilms tumour
h. Neuroblastoma
i. G6PD deficiency
j. Hereditary spherocytosis
k. Thalassaemia
l. Iron deficiency anaemia
m. Acute lymphoblastic leukaemia
n. Aplastic anaemia
o. Idiopathic thrombocytopenic purpura
p. Haemolytic anaemia

List B

a. Bone marrow aspiration
b. Blood film
c. Ferritin level
d. Hb electrophoresis
e. Osmotic fragility test
f. Red cell enzymes
g. Wrist X-ray
h. Abdominal ultrasound
i. Abdominal lymph node biopsy
j. Abdominal MRI scan
k. Endomysial antibodies
l. Mantoux test
m. Iron level and iron-binding capacity
n. Lead level
o. Urine toxicology

Case 41

1. Childhood absence epilepsy syndrome
2. Sodium valproate or ethosuximide

Childhood absence epilepsy syndrome

This is the most common form of idiopathic generalized epilepsy in children. It may occur between 4 and 11 years and usually presents as daydreaming. A typical attack occurs when the child stops what he or she is doing and does not respond for 10–20 seconds. It may be associated with eye flickering, mouthing or swallowing (automatism) and fumbling with fingers. Some children can recognize an attack but the majority cannot. The EEG is characterized by 3.5 Hz spike-wave activity. Attacks can be brought on by hyperventilation.

The treatment of choice is sodium valproate starting at 5 mg/kg/day and increasing every two weeks by 5 mg/kg/day until there are no more absences. Medication should continue for a minimum of two years. There is no need to repeat the EEG unless attacks are associated with photosensitivity.

No single gene is responsible for this condition, and genetic markers have not been fully identified. The risk for other offspring is higher than that of the normal population. Less than 5% go on to have other types of seizures or experience learning difficulties.

Case 42

1. Moderate gastro-oesophageal reflux
2. Ranitidine, domperidone and Gaviscon or Thick and Easy

Gastro-oesophageal reflux disease (GORD)

Reflux is common in infants and especially in children with neurological or developmental problems. Gastro-oesophageal reflux (GOR) is a normal phenomenon occurring in most people, especially after a meal. Gastro-oesophageal reflux disease (GORD) is acid refluxing to the lower part of the oesophagus. Symptoms in babies include pain, vomiting, arching and crying. Older children may show some discomfort and vomiting. Ambulatory 24-hour pH monitoring is the standard test to establish a diagnosis of GORD, with a sensitivity of 96% and a specificity of 95%. For positive proof of GOR, the reflux index should be more than 5% on several occasions. The condition can be classified as mild (5–10%), moderate (11–15%) or severe (16% or above).

Histamine H_2 receptor antagonists (ranitidine, cimetidine) or proton pump inhibitors (omeprazole) plus prokinetic agents (domperidone) will improve oesophageal and stomach motility. The surgical option is rarely used in a normal healthy child, as the majority (>90%) will grow out of the condition by the time they start walking and only a few may continue on medication for longer. Surgery (Nissen fundoplication) can be offered to children with severe GORD with neurological problems who do not respond to medication.

Differential diagnosis in children presenting with vomiting, wheezes and right upper lobe changes on CXR

	H-type tracheo-oesophageal fistula laryngeal cleft	Gastro-oroesophageal reflux	Hiatus hernia
Clinical features	Vomiting, recurrent aspiration, wheezes	Vomiting, recurrent aspiration, wheezes, failure to thrive	Vomiting on lying down, oesophagitis, occasional aspiration
Investigations	Cine barium swallow, bronchoscopy ± endoscopy	Barium swallow, pH study, CXR	Barium swallow, upper GIT endoscopy
Management	Surgical repair	Anti-reflux medication; consider Nissen fundoplication in severe cases and in children with cerebral palsy	Anti-reflux medication; surgical repair if not controlled by anti-reflux medication or if stenosis develops

Case 43

1. Conductive hearing loss
2. Grommet insertion

Conductive hearing loss

Conductive hearing loss occurs when sound is not conducted efficiently through the outer ear canal to the eardrum and ossicles of the middle ear. It can be caused by fluid in the middle ear from colds, allergies (serous otitis media), poor eustachian tube function, ear infection (otitis media), perforated eardrum or benign tumours. It may also be caused by external otitis, presence of a foreign body, absence or malformation of the outer ear, ear canal and middle ear, or impacted earwax. The degree of hearing loss can be assessed as follows:

- Normal range or no impairment, 0–20 dB
- Mild loss, 20–40 dB
- Moderate loss, 40–60 dB

- Severe loss, 60–80 dB
- Profound loss, 80 dB or more

Methods of checking hearing by patient age group

- Neonates can be tested using the acoustic response cradle. This is an automatic microprocessor-controlled device used to detect hearing response against a background of spontaneous activity. In high-risk groups brainstem auditory evoked response (BSAER) is the method of choice for testing hearing in neonates.
- Distraction audiometry is used as a screening test at 7–8 months of age.
- Toy discrimination test. A normal child can discriminate verbal toy stimuli at 40 dB at 3 feet. This can be applied to age 2–5 years.
- Audiometry can be applied to any child over the age of 5 years.
- Tympanometry can be applied at any age.

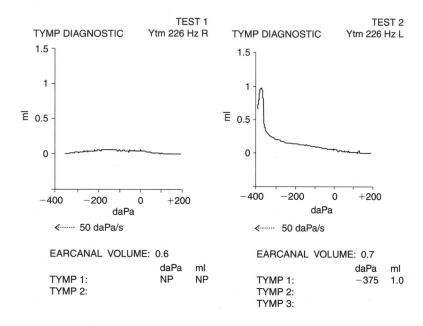

Brainstem auditory evoked response (BSAER) can be used from an early age, as a response first appears at a fetal age of 26–27 weeks.

Case 44

1. Abnormal sleep study (possible obstructive apnoea)
2. Urgent adenotonsillectomy

Obstructive sleep apnoea

Sleep apnoea is the reduction of airflow at the nose and mouth during sleep. The current treatment of choice is adenotonsillectomy (the removal of the adenoids and tonsils), due to its perceived efficacy, cost effectiveness and the relative size of adenoid and tonsil tissue in children. There is a lack of strong evidence to support the use of adenotonsillectomy in children with sleep apnoea, though there are some data to indicate that it may be beneficial; more research is required (Lim and McKean 2001). There is some debate as to the diagnosis of obstructive sleep apnoea in children, and further research and extensive diagnostic tests need to be undertaken to make an appropriate diagnosis.

Case 45

1. Ventricular tachycardia
2. Cardioversion 10 J/kg

Ventricular tachycardia

Ventricular tachycardia may cause palpitations, fatigue, chest pressure or pain, shortness of breath, fainting, light-headedness, or dizziness. It is important to note that children may not know how to describe all of the above. They may feel tired, may have 'spells' during games and need to rest, or may have no symptoms.

Ventricular tachycardia is typically secondary to structural cardiac disease, prolonged-QT syndrome, hypoxaemia, acidosis, electrolyte imbalance, and drug toxicity or poisoning. Children with signs of shock who have palpable pulses but whose condition is unstable receive synchronized cardioversion beginning at 0.5 J/kg. A lidocaine (Xylocaine) bolus (1 mg/kg) is also administered, followed by continuous infusion at a rate of 20–50 µg/kg/min. The aetiology of ventricular tachycardia must be identified and managed.

Management of ventricular tachycardia in children (Bardella 1999)

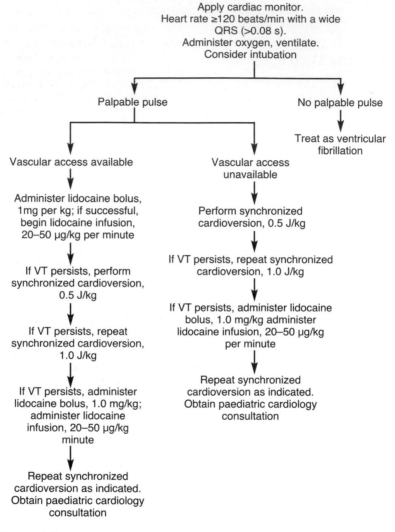

Case 46

1. Neuroblastoma
2. Bone marrow aspiration
   Abdominal MRI scan

Neuroblastoma

An abdominal mass that crosses the midline with calcification on ultrasound and no renal tissues involved is almost always a neuroblastoma arising from the adrenal gland. Phaeochromocytoma is rare.

Clinical features

Neuroblastoma usually presents as an abdominal mass. In 10% of patients, it can present with dancing eye syndrome (opsoclonus–myoclonus syndrome). This myoclonic encephalopathy is characterized by chaotic eye movements, myoclonic ataxia and encephalopathy; it may be idiopathic or occur as the result of an occult neuroblastoma. MRI of the chest and abdomen to diagnose occult neuroblastoma is indicated. Other presentations of neuroblastoma can be a lump in the neck or chest, bulging eyes, dark circles around the eyes, bone pain, swollen stomach and trouble breathing in babies, painless, bluish lumps under the skin in babies, and an inability to move a body part.

Treatments include surgery, radiation therapy, chemotherapy or a combination. ACTH or oral corticosteroids provide partial or complete relief of symptoms in 80% of patients.

Investigations

Homovanillic acid (HVA) and vanillylmandelic acid (VMA) levels in urine, and dopa, dopamine, norepinephrine (noradrenaline) and normetanephrine levels in serum are high in 90% of children with neuroblastoma. These can be assayed by mass spectrography and gas chromatography; the tests are sensitive, even if the urine or serum samples are small in quantity. A 24-hour urine collection is required to prove the diagnosis, even when mass spectrography and chromatography tests are used. The secretion of catecholamine metabolites is much higher in children with phaeochromocytoma than in those with neuroblastoma. *m*-Iodobenzylguanidine (MIBG) can be taken up by catecholamine-producing tumours and used to locate the primary tumour and metastatic lesions. Biopsy of the lesion and bone marrow trephine biopsy are the definitive diagnostic tests.

Treatment

Treatments include surgery, radiation therapy, chemotherapy or a combination of these.

Case 47

1. Idiopathic thrombocytopenic purpura
2. Bone marrow aspiration
   Blood film

Idiopathic thrombocytopenic purpura

The incidence of ITP is 50–100 new cases per million per year, and half of these cases can be in children. ITP patients can present with bruising, petechiae, nosebleeds and bleeding gums if the platelet count is below 20×10^9/l. Subarachnoid or intracerebral hemorrhage or other internal bleeding is very serious but not common, and may also occur if the platelet count is <20×10^9/l. The cause is unknown; IgG autoantibodies against the platelets can found in 60% of patients with ITP. Bone marrow aspiration is only indicated if there is no response to treatment or if the diagnosis is in doubt, or in chronic cases. The BT is long, but this is not pathognomonic. Treatment can be given if there is serious mucous membrane bleeding or CNS bleeding with very low platelets. This can be in the form of IVIG of 2 g/kg over either 48 hours or 5 days according to local protocol. Steroids also can be used as a temporary measure. Splenectomy can be used in chronic cases. Two thirds of paediatric patients will grow out of ITP without any treatment within 6 months. The remaining cases will become chronic: two thirds of these will grow out of ITP, and one third will remain chronic with mild thrombocytopenia with a platelet count of $50 \times 10^9/l$.

Case 48

1. Iron deficiency anaemia
2. Ferritin level
   Hb electrophoresis

Iron deficiency anaemia

This is the most common nutritional disorder of childhood, occurring in 12% of children in the UK. The prevalence is higher in certain ethnic minorities, namely Chinese and Afro-Caribbeans, and is almost double the national prevalence in the Pakistani, Bangladeshi and Indian populations living in the UK. There are contributing factors, which include socioeconomic status, early introduction of unmodified cows' milk into the diet with introduction of solids later, bottle-feeding for a longer period and fewer dietary supplements. Children with iron deficiency anaemia may present as having behavioural problems, repeat infections, loss of appetite, lethargy, breathlessness, increased sweating, strange food cravings (pica) such as eating dirt, and failure to thrive (short stature).

The goal of treatment is to educate parents about the dietary requirements for children. Iron supplementation is the treatment for at least 3 months, with regular follow-up by dietician, paediatrician and health visitor.

Case 49

1. Haemolytic anaemia
2. Blood film
   Osmotic fragility test

Haemolytic anaemia

Haemolysis is the premature destruction of red cells. This may lead to failure of the bone marrow to produce more erythrocytes. Symptoms depend on the cause of haemolysis and the intrinsic defect of the red cells. Haemolytic anaemia represents 5% of all anaemias. There are many types, hereditary and acquired. Hereditary types include G6PD deficiency, spherocytosis and sickle cell anaemia. Acquired haemolytic anaemias include autoimmune haemolytic anaemia and microangiopathic haemolytic anaemia.

Intravascular haemolysis may occur in patients with prosthetic heart valves, etc. Other causes may include infection, liver cirrhosis, SLE and a defect in haemoglobin, e.g. thalassaemia.

The symptoms of anaemia are similar whatever the cause. In haemolytic anaemia, the spleen can be large. This is not universal, but it is one of the common signs. The reticulocyte count is high and the unconjugated bilirubin is also high.

Treatment depends on the cause. Early blood transfusion may be needed unless there is malignancy, in which case liaison with the local oncologist is best.

Case 50

1. G6PD deficiency
2. Red cell enzymes
   Urine toxicology

Glucose-6-phosphate dehydrogenase deficiency

This is the most common enzyme deficiency affecting red cells. It occurs worldwide and can cause neonatal hyperbilirubinaemia and acute and chronic haemolysis. It is inherited as an X-linked recessive disorder and most commonly affects persons of African, Asian, Mediterranean or Middle-Eastern descent. Acute haemolysis is caused by exposure to an oxidative stressor in the form of an infection, oxidative drug or fava beans. G6PD catalyses nicotinamide adenine dinucleotide phosphate (NADP) to its reduced form, NADPH, in the pentose phosphate pathway. NADPH protects cells from oxidative damage. Because erythrocytes do not generate NADPH in any other way, they are more susceptible than other cells to destruction from oxidative stress. Acute haemolysis is self-limited, but in rare instances it can be severe enough to warrant a blood transfusion. Neonatal hyperbilirubinemia may require treatment with phototherapy or exchange transfusion to prevent kernicterus.

The gene is located on the X chromosome and there are >400 mutations. The diagnosis can be made by quantitative spectrophotometric analysis or, more commonly, by a rapid fluorescent spot test detecting the generation of NADPH from NADP.

Drugs that may cause haemolysis in patients with G6PD deficiency are dapsone, methylene blue, nalidixic acid, nitrofurantoin, phenazopyridine, primaquine and sulphonamides. Avoiding oxidative stresses will help to prevent haemolytic crises in these patients. Education of parents is very important, and joining the G6PD Deficiency Association will help them to understand this condition much better. It is a lifelong condition with constant risk of haemolysis. Splenectomy has no role, as patients are mostly asymptomatic and haemolysis is short-lived. Folic acid and iron supplements can be given during episodes of haemolysis. Genetic counselling is very important.

EMQ

For the following scenario, choose the three most likely differential diagnoses from List A and match them with the appropriate investigations from List B.

Case 51

A 10-year-old presents with generalized oedema, clubbing and tiredness. This has been going on for the last 2 months and he gets tired easily. His parents are from Slovakia and recently moved to this country.

Hb	8.7 g/dl
ESR	19 mm/h (0–10 mm/h)
WCC	11.2×10^9/l
Plt	500×10^9/l
CRP	<5 mg/l
Bilirubin	10 µmol/l
Na	132 mmol/l
K	4.1 mmol/l
U	1.3 mmol/l
Cr	60 mmol/l
Albumin	12 mmol/l
Total protein	45 mmol/l
ALP	160 mmol/l
ALT	35 mmol/l
Urine	No proteinuria or blood
Sweat test	Cl, 30 mmol/l

MRI scan of his abdomen with contrast shows thickening of small bowel loops

List A

a. Liver failure
b. Crohn's disease
c. Cystic fibrosis
d. Ulcerative colitis
e. Coeliac disease
f. Shwachman syndrome
g. Nephrotic syndrome
h. Abetalipoproteinaemia
i. Eosinophilic colitis
j. Lymphoedema
k. Small intestine TB
l. AIDS

List B

a. Upper and lower GIT endoscopy with biopsy
b. CXR
c. Mantoux test
d. DNA linkage study for Delta 508
e. 24-hour urine collection for proteinuria
f. Blood film
g. Barium swallow and follow through
h. Liver biopsy
i. Endomysial antibodies
j. HIV status
k. Kidney biopsy
l. Lymphangiography

EMQs

For the following scenarios, choose the most appropriate treatment from List B, to match the diagnosis selected from List A.

Case 52

A 14-month-old boy presents with a chest infection and an erythematous rash on his right ankle, wrists and neck. Otherwise he is a healthy young boy.

Hb	13.2 g/dl
WCC	13×10^9/l
N	7.7 (L 4.1, E 1.0, M 0.5, B 0.0)
Plt	50×10^9/l
MCV	73
Hct	<1
PT	10 s
APTT	66 s
CRP	<5 mg/l (0–8)
Total bilirubin	11 µmol/l (0–23)
Conjugated bilirubin	<1 mmol/l
ALP	250 u/l (109–272)
ALT	14 u/l (0–45)
MCHC	89
Factor VII	>2
INR	2.5

Case 53

A 5-day-old baby girl presents with lethargy, possible seizures and not feeding very well. The head ultrasound shows intracerebral bleeding. CT scan shows no subdural bleeding, but confirms the intracerebral bleeding. MRA shows no blood vessel abnormalities.

Hb	16.4 g/dl
WCC	14×10^9/l
N	7.7 (L 6.1, E 1.0, M 0.5, B 0.0)
Plt	220×10^9/l
MCV	77
Hct	<1
PT	25 s
APTT	125 s
CRP	<5 mg/l (0–8)
Total bilirubin	125 µmol/l (0–23)
Conjugated bilirubin	<1 mmol/l
ALP	210 u/l (109–272)
ALT	19 u/l (0–45)
MCHC	103
INR	3.1

Case 54

A 13-year-old girl presents with a purpuric rash and multiple bruises on her legs and forearms. She is well, with no organomegaly or large lymph nodes.

Hb	12.7 g/dl
WCC	11×10^9/l
N	6.7 (L 4.1, E 1.0, M 0.5, B 0.0)
Plt	240×10^9/l
PT	10 s
BT	10 min
APTT	90 s
INR	1.1

Blood film shows no lymphoblasts, and anisocytosis

Case 55

A 2-year-old boy presents with bruises on his legs, back and forearms.

Hb	8.6 g/dl
WCC	4.6 × 10⁹/l
N	1.7 (L 2.1, E 1.0, M 0.5, B 0.0)
Plt	20 × 10⁹/l
MCV	66
Hct	<1
PT	10 s
APTT	86 s
CRP	12 mg/l (0–8)
Total bilirubin	15 µmol/l (0–23)
Conjugated bilirubin	<1 mmol/l
ALP	2400 u/l (109–272)
ALT	18 u/l (0–45)
MCHC	88
Factor VIII	Low <2
INR	1.2

Bone marrow shows hypoplasia and featureless cells, with no lymphoblasts or myeloblasts

List A

a. Hodgkin lymphoma
b. Acute lymphoblastic leukaemia
c. Wiskott–Aldrich syndrome
d. Henoch–Schönlein purpura
e. Haemophilia A
f. TAR syndrome
g. Aplastic anaemia
h. Haemophilia B
i. Haemorrhagic disease of the newborn
j. Non-Hodgkin lymphoma
k. Idiopathic thrombocytopenic purpura
l. Disseminated malignancy

List B

a. Blood film
b. Cranial MRI
c. Analgesia for pain and supportive therapy
d. Bone marrow aspiration
e. Factor XI level
f. IM vitamin K injection
g. Factor VII level
h. Bone marrow transplant
i. Liver biopsy
j. INR
k. Clotting profile
l. Thymic scan

EMQs

For the following scenarios, choose the most likely diagnosis from List A, and two added investigations to help in diagnosis from List B. From List C, select three steps of your initial management.

Case 56

A 5-day-old baby girl presented with lethargy and tachycardia of 190/min. She was sleepy with BP 50/35. Her weight had dropped from 2.560 kg to 2.350 kg.

Hb	20.5 g/dl
WCC	17×10^9/l
Plt	180×10^9/l
MCV	80
MCHC	107
CRP	<5 mg/l (0–8)
Total bilirubin	156 μmol/l (0–23)
ALT	19 u/l (0–45)
ALP	130 u/l (109–272)
Albumin	32 g/l (35–50)
Na	166 mmol/l
K	3.7 mmol/l
U	22 mmo/l
Cr	109 mmol/l
Ca	2.00 mmol/l
Corrected Ca	2.11 mmol/l
Mg	0.9 mmol/l
P	1.71 mmol/l

Case 57

A 3-year-old presented with high temperature, abdominal pain and vomiting.

Na	137 mmol/l
Albumin	44 g/l (35–50)
K	3.7 mmol/l
U	7.8 mmo/l
Cr	90 mmol/l
Ca	2.00 mmol/l
Corrected Ca	2.20 mmol/l
Mg	0.8 mmol/l
P	1.55 mmol

Urine microscopy <100 WCC, no nitrates, 200 red cells and +protein
Renal ultrasound shows right multidysplastic kidneys and upper polar scar on left kidney

Case 58

A 10-year-old is admitted to hospital one day after returning home from holiday in the USA. He developed diarrhoea 2 days before leaving the USA, with some blood in his stools.

Hb	7.8 g/dl
CRP	35 mg/l (0–8)
WCC	12 × 10⁹/l
N	6.7 (L 5.1, E 1.0, M 0.5, B 0.0)
Plt	220 × 10⁹/l
MCV	77 fl
MCHC	89 fl
PT	10 s
APTT	80 s
Total bilirubin	10 µmol/l (0–23)
ALP	180 u/l (109–272)
ALT	18 u/l (0–45)
INR	1.6
Na	131 mmol/l
Albumin	32 g/l (35–50)
K	5.7 mmol/l
U	35 mmol/l
Cr	175 mmol/l
Ca	2.10 mmol/l
Corrected Ca	2.32 mmol/l
Mg	0.9 mmol/l
P	1.40 mmol

Blood film showed ghost cells, microcytic, hypochromic anaemia, aniso-cytosis

Case 59

A 12-day-old baby boy was born at 25 weeks' gestation. He was venti-lated for 4 days and since then has been on CPAP. He is still on TPN and managing only 1 ml of expressed breast milk every 2 hours as there is bile aspirate and he has a distended abdomen.

Hb	12.5 g/dl
WCC	7 × 10⁹/l
N	4.7 (L2.1, E 1.0, M 0.5, B 0.0)
Plt	220 × 10⁹/l
MCV	80 fl
Hct	<1
CRP	<5 mg/l (0–8)
ALP	190 u/l (109–272)
ALT	25 u/l (0–45
Total bilirubin	75 µmol/l (0–23)
Conjugated bilirubin	<1 mmol/l
MCHC	107
PT	10 s

APTT	90 s
INR	1.0
Na	129 mmol/l
Albumin	28 g/l (35–50)
K	5.8 mmol/l
U	19 mmol/l
Cr	200 mmol/l
Ca	1.90 mol/l

Urine output is 0.3 ml/h/kg/day

Case 60

A 6-year-old boy presents with swelling of his face, scrotum and abdomen.

Na	133 mmol/l
Albumin	21 g/l (35–50)
K	3.8 mmol/l
U	3.5 mmol/l
Cr	55 mmol/l
Ca	1.90 mmol/l

LFT, TFT are within normal range

Urine output is 3 ml/h/kg/day, with no hyaline casts and no blood or nitrites

List A

a. Acute renal failure
b. Acute glomerulonephritis
c. Nephrotic syndrome
d. Haemolytic uraemic syndrome
e. UTI
f. Polycystic renal disease
g. Chronic renal failure
h. Hypernatraemic dehydration
i. Liver failure
j. SIADH
k. Pre-renal failure
l. Reflux nephropathy

List B

a. Renal ultrasound
b. Urine culture
c. 24-hour urine collection for protein
d. 24-hour urine collection for creatinine–calcium ratio
e. DMSA scan
f. MCUG
g. Stool culture
h. IVU

i.   C3 and C4
j.   Renal biopsy
k.   Indirect MAG3
l.   Monitor urinary output

List C

a.   Peritoneal renal dialysis
b.   IV maintenance fluid + deficit over 48 hours with 0.9% NaCl + 5% glucose
c.   IV maintenance fluid + deficit over 48 hours with 0.45% NaCl + 5% glucose
d.   IV antibiotics
e.   Haemodialysis
f.   Oral prednisolone 80 mg/m²/day for 4 weeks, 60 mg/m²/day for 4 weeks, 40 mg/m²/day for 4 weeks, 20 mg/m²/day for 4 weeks
g.   Start prednisolone 2 mg/kg/day for 4 weeks and reduce slowly over 4 weeks
h.   Refer to a nephrologist
i.   Give prophylactic antibiotics and refer to a nephrologist
j.   IV albumin infusion of 4.8%
k.   IV albumin infusion of 20%
l.   Supportive therapy of nutrition
m.   Refer to a tertiary centre
n.   Restrict fluid to 300 ml/m²/day and refer to a nephrologist
o.   Prophylactic trimethoprim

Case 51

1. Crohn's disease
   Coeliac disease
   Small intestine TB
2. Upper and lower GIT endoscopy with biopsy
   Endomysial antibodies
   Mantoux test, CXR

Hypoalbuminaemia

Albumin comprises 75–80% of normal plasma colloid oncotic pressure and 50% of protein content. Albumin can transport various substances, including ions, bilirubin, fatty acids, metals, hormones and exogenous drugs. In hypoalbuminaemia, transport of all of these can be affected.

The common causes of low albumin in children include:

a. Nutritional status (poor protein intake, e.g. starvation)
b. Increased excretion of albumin via the kidney (nephrotic syndrome), liver (liver cirrhosis or failure), heart (congestive heart failure), GIT (inflammatory bowel diseases), extensive burns, lymphatic blockage, sarcoma, amyloidosis and tuberculosis

Treatment should focus on the underlying cause. Albumin infusion may be harmful and can increase mortality. If fluid restriction is not helping to reduce the oedema and albumin leakage continues, then colloids can be used. There is limited evidence for the use of albumin infusion in such cases.

Case 52

1. Wiskott–Aldrich syndrome
2. Clotting profile
   Thymic scan

Wiskott–Aldrich syndrome (WAS)

WAS has characteristic features that include:

a. Thrombocytopenia (increased tendency to bleed)
b. Recurrent bacterial, viral and fungal infections (both humoral and cellular immunity are affected)
c. Eczema of the skin

It is inherited as an X-linked recessive trait, and the patient may present with all features but sometimes with only two, and in different combinations. The *WAS* gene is located on the Xp11.22–23 region of the X chromosome. A male child of a female carrier has a 50% chance of being affected; a female child has a 50% chance of being a carrier. A reduced number of platelets of small size are a characteristic feature in all patients with WAS. Patients usually present with petechial rashes. Malignancies can occur in young children, as well as in adolescents and adults with WAS. Most of these malignancies involve B-lymphocytes, resulting in lymphoma or leukaemia. The diagnosis can be made by looking at the platelet count (low) and blood film, which will show platelets that are small. The usual vaccine response is absent. The diagnosis is usually confirmed by demonstrating a decrease or absence of the WAS protein (WASp) in blood cells or by the presence of a mutation within the *WAS* gene.

Treatment should be supportive until a matched donor can be found. Prophylactic antibiotics and immunoglobulins should be given on a regular basis, treating infection rapidly as well as preventing blood loss.

Case 53

1. Haemorrhagic disease of the newborn
2. IM vitamin K injection

Haemorrhagic disease of the newborn

Haemorrhagic disease of the newborn (HDN) is due to vitamin K deficiency. Vitamin K is required for the production of clotting factors II, VII, IX and X. It is present in some plants and is also synthesized by some *Escherichia coli* in the gut. All newborn infants have low levels of vitamin K and are at risk of developing HDN. The body has a very limited ability to store vitamin K.

There are risk factors that increase the incidence of HDN: children who are entirely breastfed have a 20 times greater risk than those who receive formula milk, due to the low level of vitamin K in breast milk and also the low levels of bacteria that help to synthesize vitamin K in the guts of breastfed babies. Several drugs, such as isoniazid, rifampicin, anticoagulants and anticonvulsant agents, when taken by the mother, put the infant at risk of developing early HDN. Warm environmental temperatures also predispose babies to developing late HDN. Unsuspected liver disease, especially α_1-antitrypsin deficiency, increases the risk, as does malabsorption of fat-soluble vitamins due to diarrhoea, coeliac disease or cystic fibrosis.

All newborn babies should receive oral vitamin K; in some countries, it is given intramuscularly (IM). The putative risk of malignancy with IM vitamin K is not proven, as larger studies have failed to substantiate this. If HDN occurs, subcutaneous vitamin K should be given as soon as possible. Babies with intracranial bleeding need fresh frozen plasma in addition to vitamin K.

A Cochrane review concluded that a single dose (1.0 mg) of IM vitamin K after birth is effective in the prevention of classic HDN. Either IM or oral (1.0 mg) vitamin K prophylaxis improves biochemical indices of coagulation status at 1–7 days. Neither IM nor oral vitamin K has been tested in randomized trials with respect to effect on late HDN. Oral vitamin K, either single- or multiple-dose, has not been tested in randomized trials for its effect on either classic or late HDN. In babies born before 32 weeks' gestation, 0.5 mg would appear to be sufficient (Puckett and Offringa 2000).

Case 54

1. Henoch–Schönlein purpura
2. Analgesia for pain and supportive therapy

Henoch–Schönlein purpura

Henoch–Schönlein purpura (HSP) is a type of vasculitis, an inflammatory response within the blood vessel. HSP is an IgA-mediated small vessel vasculitis. It is caused by an abnormal response of the immune system, the mechanism of which is unknown. It affects children of any age and usually appears 2 weeks after URTI. The initial presentation may be with a purpuric rash affecting the lower limbs and sometimes the upper limbs around the elbows, and occasionally the ear lobes. The symptoms can be a combination of any or all of the following: abdominal pain, angioedema, joint pain, purpura, vomiting, diarrhoea and nausea. Infection, bleeding disorder and intestinal obstruction (intussusception) must be excluded. Supportive treatment for pain should be given, checking urine for blood for the first 6 weeks. Steroids are rarely helpful and HSP resolves spontaneously. A randomized placebo-controlled study of 40 children with HSP was conducted, in which 21 received prednisone within 7 days of disease onset and 19 received placebo. Early treatment did not reduce the risk of renal or GIT involvement (Rosenblum and Winter 1987).

Case 55

1. Aplastic anaemia
2. Bone marrow transplant

Aplastic anaemia

Aplastic anaemia is a syndrome of bone marrow failure characterized by peripheral pancytopenia and marrow hypoplasia. Fanconi anaemia is one of the causes of aplastic anaemia. Other causes can be divided into congenital or inherited (20%), e.g. dyskeratosis congenita, cartilage–hair hypoplasia, Pearson syndrome, amegakaryocytic thrombocytopenia (thrombocytopenia–absent radius (TAR) syndrome), Shwachman–Diamond syndrome, Dubowitz syndrome, Diamond–Blackfan syndrome and familial aplastic anaemia. Acquired causes (80%) include, idiopathic factors, infectious causes (e.g. hepatitis viruses, EBV, HIV, parvovirus and mycobacteria), toxic exposure to radiation and chemicals (e.g.

benzene and drugs such as chloramphenicol, phenylbutazone and gold), transfusional GVHD, orthotopic liver transplantation for fulminant hepatitis, and eosinophilic fasciitis.

Fanconi anaemia

Fanconi anaemia is inherited as an autosomal recessive trait; it has a higher prevalence in males than in females.

Clinical features

This is one of the DNA repair disorders associated with a high risk of malignancy. It can present in different ways, e.g. with aplastic anaemia, leukaemia, leukopenia, thrombocytopenia and tumours. About half of the patients will have hyperpigmented patches, 'café-au-lait' spots, microsomy, microcephaly, thumb anomalies, other skeletal anomalies, micro-ophthalmia and mental retardation.

Patients often present with low platelets or low WCC before pancytopenia, which always starts mildly and then becomes severe. The red cells are macrocytic, there is raised HbF, and the bone marrow initially shows areas of hypercellularity, which disappear as bone marrow failure occurs.

Diagnosis and treatment

The diagnosis can be made by identification of breakage, gaps and rearrangement in the DNA of stimulated lymphocytes. The androgen oxymetholone is used to prolong survival; virilization and stunting are two major side effects.

The only curative treatment is allogeneic bone marrow transplantation. Because of the increased susceptibility of patients with DNA repair defects, special pretransplantation conditioning regimens are employed, using low-dose alkylating agents and low-dose (or no) irradiation. Malignancy will develop sooner or later in 15% of patients. Half of these will have myeloid-type leukaemia and the other half will have liver or other tumours. Androgens may exacerbate the genetic risk of liver disease.

Case 56

1. Hypernatraemic dehydration
2. Renal ultrasound
3. IV maintenance fluid + deficit over 48 hours (0.9% NaCl and 5% glucose)

Hypernatraemia

This is defined as a serum sodium level of >145 mmol/l, which is due to either loss of free water or increased intake of hypertonic solutions. It may be caused by the following three mechanisms, either alone or together:

- Pure water depletion (e.g. diabetes insipidus)
- Water depletion exceeding sodium depletion (e.g. diarrhoea)
- Sodium excess (e.g. salt poisoning)

There are many causes of hypernatraemia, the most common of which are hypovolaemic, e.g. diarrhoea and euvolaemic-like diabetes insipidus. Treatment should be aimed towards the cause, which should be ascertained from history and examination plus targeted blood tests or imaging.

Hypernatraemia should be corrected over 48 hours. The level of sodium should be monitored closely and not allowed to decrease by more than 1–2 mmol/l every 3–4 hours. Fluid correction should be done over 48 hours using 0.45% and 5% glucose.

Case 57

1. Reflux nephropathy
2. Indirect MAG3
3. Prophylactic trimethoprim and referral to a nephrologist

Reflux nephropathy

There is a small and scarred kidney associated with vesicoureteric reflux (VUR). Reflux nephropathy is an important cause of end-stage renal failure. It may cause hypertension, proteinuria and decreased renal function when scarring is extensive. Renal scarring was seen in more than 30% of cases in children with VUR. Children under the age of 5 years who have UTI are more prone to VUR and reflux nephropathy. Changes in guidelines for investigation of infants and children who present with UTI are in progress. NICE (2007) have produced new guidelines for children with UTI. There is much debate about the use of prophylactic antibiotics, as well as the need for extensive investigation for VUR and scarring. KUB US is the key investigation after a proven UTI. If the results are abnormal, further testing consists of either MCUG in a child under 6 months or indirect MAG3 followed by DMSA in children under or over 6 months. If no scarring is visible on US, the child can be discharged. Local protocols should be followed at all times.

Case 58

1. Haemolytic uraemic syndrome
2. Monitor urinary output
3. Restrict fluid to 300 ml/m^2/day and refer

Haemolytic uraemic syndrome

Haemolytic uraemic syndrome (HUS) is the most common cause of acute renal failure in young children. It is characterized by the triad of microangiopathic anaemia, thrombocytopenia and renal failure.

Causes

The cause is unknown, but HUS can be associated with bacterial or viral infection of the GIT or respiratory system. HUS can also be associated with SLE, malignant hypertension and endotoxaemia.

Pathophysiology

There is endothelial injury. The microangiopathic anaemia results from mechanical damage to the red cells as they pass through damaged vasculature. Thrombocytopenia is due to intravascular platelet adhesion or damage.

Types of HUS

The type of HUS that is epidemic and occurs in young children following gastroenteritis has a good prognosis. The sporadic form without known cause that occurs in older children may lead to chronic renal failure and early death.

Clinical features

HUS mostly occurs 1–2 weeks after gastroenteritis, with pallor, lethargy, dark urine, weakness and oliguria.

SLE can be associated with microangiopathic anaemia. Bilateral renal vein thrombosis may follow gastroenteritis. It may present with microangiopathic anaemia, low platelets and acute renal failure with large kidneys – a characteristic feature of renal vein thrombosis.

Management

Renal failure can be managed conservatively, and early management with frequent peritoneal dialysis or haemodialysis will give the best chance of recovery. Plasmapheresis, anticoagulant and fresh frozen plasma are used as part of the management; the results are not good as frequent peritoneal dialysis or haemodialysis.

Prognosis

The prognosis in the epidemic form is good; the sporadic form may lead to chronic renal failure. With aggressive management of acute renal failure, >90% of patients with HUS will survive the acute phase and the majority of these recover normal renal function.

Case 59

1. Pre-renal failure
2. Measure renal output
3. Supportive

Acute pre-renal failure

Causes

Pre-renal	Renal	Post-renal
Hypovolaemia, e.g. DKA, haemorrhage, gastroenteritis	Hypovolaemia	Posterior urethral valves
Peripheral vasodilatation, e.g. sepsis	Disease of kidney, e.g. acute glomerulonephritis	Crystals (uric acid)
Cardiac failure	HUS, cortical necrosis	Neurogenic bladder
Bilateral renal vessel occlusion	Surgical accident	Severe UTI
GIT obstruction	Nephrotoxins	Calculus
	Myoglobinuria	Ureterocele
	Haemoglobinuria	Tumours
		Trauma

Diagnosis

Features of renal failure are oliguria, oedema, acidotic breathing and drowsiness. Acute hypertensive encephalopathy may occur.

	Pre-renal	Renal
Na (urine)	<20 mmol/l	>30 mmol/l
U:P osmolality ratio	>1:1.5	<1:1
U:P urea ratio	>10	<10
Urine osmolality	>400 mmol/kg	<400 mmol/kg
U:P creatinine ratio	>20	<20

Case 60

1. Nephrotic syndrome
2. 24-hour urine collection for protein
3. Oral prednisolone 80 mg/m²/day for 4 weeks, 60 mg/m²/day for 4 weeks, 40 mg/m²/day for 4 weeks, 20 mg/m²/day for 4 weeks

Treatment of nephrotic syndrome

Corticosteroids remain the first line of treatment for nephrotic syndrome on first presentation. The regimen is different from place to place. The current recommendation is that the longer the course of corticosteroids, the less risk there is of early relapse, i.e. 4 months on corticosteroids, starting with oral prednisolone 60 mg/m^2/day for 4 weeks, 40 mg/m^2/day for 4 weeks, 20 mg/m^2/day for 4 weeks and then reducing by 5 mg every week.

Non-steroidal treatment of nephrotic syndrome

The authors of the Cochrane review (Hodson et al 2001) identified 26 studies (1173 children). Cyclophosphamide (response rate 0.44, 95% CI 0.26–0.73) and chlorambucil (response rate 0.15, 95% CI 0.02–0.95) significantly reduced the relapse risk at 6–12 months compared with prednisone alone. There was no difference in relapse risk at 2 years between chlorambucil and cyclophosphamide (response rate 1.31, 95% CI 0.80–2.13). There was no difference at one year between intravenous and oral cyclophosphamide (response rate 0.99, 95% CI 0.76–1.29). Ciclosporin was as effective as cyclophosphamide (response rate 1.07, 95% CI 0.48–2.35) and chlorambucil (response rate 0.82, 95% CI 0.44–1.53), and levamisole (response rate 0.43, 95% CI 0.27–0.68) was more effective than steroids alone but the effects were not sustained once treatment was stopped. There was no difference in the risk for relapse between mycophenolate mofetil and ciclosporin (response rate 5.00, 95% CI 0.68–36.66), but CI were large. Mizoribine and azathioprine were no more effective than placebo or prednisone alone in maintaining remission.

EMQ

For the following scenario, choose two differential diagnoses from List A and match them with the most appropriate investigation related to each diagnosis from List B.

Case 61

A 5-year-old boy presents with a history of recurrent skin infections. He has required drainage of abscess on two occasions. There are no other concerns about him.

Hb	13 g/dl
WCC	4.9×10^9/l
N	2.3 (L 1.7, E 0.4, M 0.5, B 0.0)
Plt	290×10^9/l
Blood film	mild neutrophilia
CRP	<5 mg/l (0–8)
Total bilirubin	8 µmol/l (0–23)
ALP	146 mmol/l (109–272)
ALT	13 mmol/l (0–45)
Albumin	39 g/l (35–50)
ESR	1 mm/h (0–10)
IgG	11.2 g/l (4.9–16.1)
IgA	1.51 g/l (0.4–2)
IgM	1.31 g/l (0.05–0.2)
IgG subclasses	
IgG1	8.66 g/l (3.6–7.3)
IgG2	2.06 g/l (1.4–4.5)
IgG3	0.65 g/l (0.3–1.1)
IgG4	1.09 g/l (0–1)

Skin swab shows *Staphylococcus aureus*

List A

a. AIDS
b. Cyclic neutropenia
c. Chronic granulomatous disease
d. Severe combined immune deficiency
e. DiGeorge syndrome
f. Wiskott–Aldrich syndrome
g. Agammaglobulinaemia
h. Colonization of the skin with *Staphylococcus aureus*

List B

a. Bone marrow aspiration
b. Nitroblue tetrazolium test (NBT)
c. Dihydroamine test
d. CD4:CD8 ratio
e. HIV antibodies
f. Repeat blood film during infection
g. FISH chromosomal study
h. CXR
i. Nasal and skin swabs

Case 62

A boy was born at 32 weeks' gestation to a mother with type 1 diabetes. He was ventilated from day 1 to day 7 and was then on NCPAP of 7 cm water pressure in 40–55% O_2 until day 27. He was transferred to a tertiary paediatric hospital for further testing.

He was oedematous for the first 7 days and had wide-spaced nipples, low-set ears, a short neck, dilated cardiomyopathy and stridor. Positive genetic testing showed the presence of the *PTPN11* gene. Latest results are as follows:

Capillary blood gas

Po_2	5.05 kPa
Pco_2	8.12 kPa
pH	7.30
HCO^{-3}	23 kPa
BE	4.4
ALP	600 IU/l
ALT	13 IU/l
Albumin	27 g/l
U	3.5 mmol/l
Cr	38 µmol/l
Bilirubin	17 µmol/l
Na	136 mmol/l
K	4.4 mmol/l
Ca	2.19 mmol/l
PO_4	1.21 mmol/l
Mg	0.93 mmol/l

1. **What is the most likely diagnosis?**
   a. Turner syndrome
   b. DiGeorge syndrome
   c. Noonan syndrome
   d. Aicardi syndrome
   e. Williams syndrome

2. **What other two investigations would you perform?**
   a. Echocardiography
   b. Bronchoscopy
   c. CXR
   d. Renal ultrasound
   e. Lung biopsy

Case 63

A heart murmur is noticed in a 6-year-old girl and cardiac catheterization is performed.

Pressure	(mmHg)	O$_2$ saturation (%)
SVC	5	70
RA	5	73
RV	60/5	86
PA	60/20	85
LA	11	93
LV	103/60	91
AO	103/60	92

1. What is the diagnosis?
2. Should the child be excluded from exercise at school?
3. How should this child be followed up?

Case 64

A 7-year-old boy presents with a history of difficulty in breathing over a period of 3 days. RR is 27, Sao$_2$ 90–91 in air, BP 90/65 and temperature 37.8 °C, and there is no lymphadenopathy. Chest movement and air entry on the right side are reduced, with dull percussion notes. Spleen removed at 3 years of age.

Hb	11 g/dl
WCC	26.2 × 10^9/l (N 85%, L 11%, E 2%, M 1.3%)
Plt	265 × 10^9/l

Pleural aspirate performed for diagnostic and treatment purposes:

Protein	37 mmol/l
Lymphocytes	+
Organisms	Gram-positive cocci
Cytology	Normal cells (neutrophilia)
AAFB	Negative
Culture	Negative

1. What is the most likely organism causing the pleural effusion?
   a. *Pseudomonas aeruginosa*
   b. Mycoplasma
   c. *Streptococcus pneumoniae*
   d. *Haemophilus influenzae*
   e. Mycobacteria

2. What is the treatment for this case?
   a. Chest drain
   b. IV antibiotics for 7 days
   c. Pleurodesis
   d. Chest physiotherapy
   e. Intrapleural thromboplastin

Case 65

These are the results following an ITT, TRH and LHRH in a short 12-year-old boy.

	Time (min)					
	0	20	30	60	90	120
Glucose (mmol/l)	5.2	1.8	5.9	7.4	8.6	8.8
Cortisol (nmol/l)	507	—	1058	1378	1033	778
GH (mU/l)	16	8.2	7.1	6.1	4.0	13
TSH (mU/l)	2.0	13	—	8.4	—	—
FSH (u/l)	0.6	—	2.6	3.6	—	—
LH (u/l)	1	—	5.6	4.8	—	—

1. What is the diagnosis?
2. Which one further investigation is indicated?
3. Suggest two underlying causes.

Case 66

These are the lung functions of a child having difficulty in breathing:

	Predicted	Measured	%
FVC (l)	2.41	1.91	79
FEV$_1$ (l)	2.19	1.76	81
FEV$_1$/FVC (%)	91	92	2
PEF (l/min)	314	275	88
FEF% (l/s)	1.29	1.14	89

1. What disease does the child suffer from?
2. What is the most likely cause?

Case 67

A baby born at 26 weeks' gestation was ventilated from the age of 2 minutes and Curosurf given for HMD. On day 3, the ventilator settings were as follows: rate 50/min, iT 0.45 s, PIP/PEEP 18/4, FiO$_2$ 35%.

UAC blood gas
pH	7.34
P_{CO_2}	5.6 kPa
P_{O_2}	6.2 kPa
BE	−3.1
MAP	32 mmHg without inotropic support

4 hours later, following the last gas, the O$_2$ requirement increased to 70%, and the baby became bradycardic. An arterial blood gas was taken at this time and showed the following:

pH	7.21
P_{CO_2}	8.80 kPa
P_{O_2}	3.06 kPa
BE	−9.0

1. **Find the possible cause and match it with the appropriate bedside action from the following:**

   1. Pneumothorax
   2. Sepsis
   3. Necrotizing enterocolitis
   4. Dislodged tube
   5. IVH
   6. Seizures
   7. Blocked ETT
   8. Apnoea of prematurity
   9. Pulmonary haemorrhage
   10. Aspiration

   a. LP
   b. Chest illumination
   c. CXR
   d. Cranial ultrasound
   e. Echocardiography
   f. Cerebral flow monitoring
   g. Abdominal X-ray
   h. Full septic screen

2. **What is the abnormality on the blood gas?**
   a. Respiratory acidosis
   b. Respiratory alkalosis
   c. Metabolic acidosis
   d. Compensatory respiratory acidosis
   e. Metabolic alkalosis

3. **How would you manage this baby?**
   a. Change the ventilator set-up
   b. Inform a senior colleague
   c. Insert a chest drain
   d. Inform the parents
   e. Repeat CXR

Case 68

The following are the results of cardiac catheterization in a 3-day-old boy with congenital heart disease:

	O₂ saturation (%)	Pressure (mmHg)
PA	83	24
PV	97	
LA	95	10
LV	89	104/10
AO	82	79

1. What is the diagnosis?
2. What is the current treatment?

Case 69

This is the family tree of a family with an inherited disorder and a mutation in a gene located on chromosome 7.

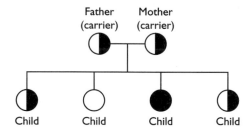

1. **What is the inheritance?**
    a. Autosomal recessive
    b. X-linked recessive
    c. Autosomal dominant
    d. X-linked dominant
    e. None of the above

2. **What is the sibling risk of getting the same condition?**
    a. 25%
    b. 50%
    c. 100%
    d. 10%
    e. None

3. **What further three investigations are available to diagnose this condition?**
    a. DNA study
    b. Sweat test
    c. Lung biopsy
    d. Skin biopsy
    e. Neonatal screen

Case 70

An ataxic 3-year-old girl is seen in the paediatric neurology clinic. Investigations include:

FBC + film	Normal
MRI	Generalized brain atrophy
Amino acids and organic acids	Normal
Alpha-fetoprotein	25 mmol/l (10–30 mmol/l)
Plasma lactate	2.1 normal
CSF lactate	1.2 normal
Very long-chain fatty acids	Normal
Nerve conduction study and EMG	Normal
Urinary VMA	500 mmol/l (30–80 mmol/l)

1. **What is the diagnosis?**
    a. Ataxia telangiectasia
    b. Friedreich ataxia
    c. Neuroblastoma
    d. Vitamin B$_{12}$ deficiency
    e. Familial hereditary ataxia

2. **Which two other clinical signs should be looked for?**
    a. Telangiectasia of the eyes
    b. Absent reflexes in lower limbs
    c. Nystagmus
    d. Hepatosplenomegaly
    e. High blood pressure

3. **List three other investigations:**
    a. 24-hour urinary collection for VMA
    b. DNA breakage study
    c. Bone marrow biopsy
    d. Liver biopsy
    e. Abdominal ultrasound

Case 61

1. Colonization of the skin with *Staphylococcus aureus*
   Chronic granulomatous disease
2. Skin and nasal swabs
   Nitroblue tetrazolium test (NBT)

Colonization with *Staphylococcus aureus*

Staphylococci are Gram-positive spherical bacteria that can be isolated on culture from the nose and skin of normal humans. The carrier status for the general population is varied. Children who are colonized with *S. aureus* usually present with repeated skin infections. These usually start as small erythematous areas, which within two days become abscesses. If antibiotics are not given, the infection will spread rapidly and may lead to scalded skin syndrome. Children who present on two or more occasions should have a blood test including immunoglobulin and IgG subclass levels, CRP, and response to vaccination especially *Haemophilus influenzae* and pneumococcus (*Streptococcus pneumoniae*). An NBT should be performed, as should swabbing of the nose and throat as well as the lesions.

Children whose skin is colonized should receive local and oral antibiotics after discussion with the microbiologist. Treatment is described below.

Suggested first-line investigations for children suspected of having immune deficiency

Disease	Presentation	Investigations
Hypogammaglobulinaemia IgM, IgA, IgG subclass deficiency	Pneumonia, otitis media, osteomyelitis, meningitis	IGs, IgG subclasses, absent thymus, FBC + differential, CH50
Hyper-IgE syndrome		
Deficient cellular immunity (e.g. AIDS)	Frequent viral infections, muco-cutaneous candidiasis, PCP	FBC + differential, CH50, lymphocyte subset, absent tonsils
Pyridoxase deficiency (chronic granulomatous disease)	Frequent abscesses (liver, lung and neck)	NBT, neutrophil function
Cyclic neutropenia	Skin sepsis and otitis media	Timed WCC with differential
Complement defect	Respiratory, GIT infections and recurrent meningitis	Defect on alternative pathway or deficiency in terminal component
Immotile cilia syndrome	Pneumonia, sinusitis, bronchiectasis	Bronchoscopy

S. *aureus*-colonized patients can be treated as follows. The treatment is primarily mupirocin cream applied to the nose three times per day for 5 days, with repeat cultures 2 days later to determine if treatment has been successful. The child with a history of relatively severe and recurrent infection still needs an immune work-up.

Case 62

1. Noonan syndrome
2. Echocardiography
   CXR

Noonan syndrome (NS)

NS is an autosomal dominant condition, and mapping of the genome has identified the mutation on the *PTPN11* gene at chromosome 12q24.1. It is not the only gene involved, but testing for this gene should be carried out. The most common features associated with Noonan syndrome are pulmonary valvular stenosis in half the patients and ASD in 10%; VSD is less common. Undescended testicles, webbed neck, lack of sexual development, poor coordination, motor delay, learning difficulties and speech delay are other features commonly associated with NS. Skeletal-like osteoporosis is less common, but easy bruising can be seen early due to clotting factor problems with combined coagulation deficiencies. Short stature is almost universal. Less frequent are joint contractures or tightness, joint hyperextensibility or looseness, and excess skin on the back of the neck with low hairline at the nape of the neck. The eyes are wide-set with diamond-shaped eyebrows, and there is a small, upturned nose. In most cases, the ears are low-set, and over 90% of cases have backward rotated ears with a thick helix. A deeply grooved philtrum can be seen in almost every case. Poor tongue control and hirsutism are less frequent.

Case 63

1. Ventricular septal defect with increased pulmonary pressure
2. Yes
3. Echocardiography every 6 months with ECG and/or CXR; growth assessment

Ventricular septal defect (VSD)

The results of cardiac catheterization show that the blood in the right ventricle has higher oxygen content than that in the right atrium. The oxygen content of blood in the pulmonary artery is slightly higher. If the VSD is large then the pulmonary blood flow is high, with equal systemic and pulmonary pressures.

Normal values for cardiac catheterization

	RA	LA	RV	LV	PA	Aorta
Sao$_2$	65%	99%	65%	98%	65%	97%
Pressure	4 mmHg	6 mmHg	25/4 mmHg	75/6 mmHg	25/15 mmHg	75/7 mmHg

Approximately 40–50% of small VSDs close spontaneously before the first birthday. Spontaneous closure is less common in moderate and large defects, even if the VSD becomes smaller as the child grows up. A small percentage of patients (2%) are at risk of developing endocarditis. Prophylactic antibiotics are necessary in patients who need dental surgery, tonsillectomy, adenoidectomy, or instrumentation of the genitourinary and gastrointestinal system. This risk is independent of the size of the VSD.

There is no restriction on the physical activity of children with VSD if there is no evidence of pulmonary hypertension. They should be allowed to participate in sport activity according to their ability. A few patients develop elevated pulmonary arterial pressure as a result of an increase in pulmonary blood flow if the repair is not performed early in large VSDs.

Management

Medical management in patients with large VSDs consists of treating chest infection, adequate nutrition with regular follow-up, and diuretics if required. If this fails, then surgery should be performed early rather than late. The prognosis is excellent following surgery.

Case 64

1. *Streptococcus pneumoniae*
2. a, b, d, e

Lobar pneumonia

Approximately 1–2% of patients with splenectomy are in danger of developing fatal sepsis with *S. pneumoniae* and *H. influenzae*. The pneumococcal vaccine and prophylactic antibiotics (penicillin) should be given to these patients. Less than 5% of patients may develop secondary 'leukaemic' changes.

Treatment for pleural effusion as a complication of lobar pneumonia includes inserting a chest drain until there is no more drainage for 24 hours, intravenous antibiotics for 7 days according to sensitivity from pleural fluid culture, chest physiotherapy, and in some cases intrapleural thromboplastin. The child should be followed up and CXR repeated after 4–6 weeks.

Case 65

1. Partial growth hormone insufficiency
2. CT scan with contrast or MRI of the brain
3. Pituitary tumour, septo-optic dysplasia

Growth hormone (GH) insufficiency

A normal GH response is accepted as >15–20 mU/l, depending on the assay. A partial response with levels <7 mU/l is a GH deficiency.

Other causes of short stature should be excluded prior to performing a GH provocation test. These include chronic illness, chronic renal failure and renal tubular acidosis. Additional endocrine causes such as hypothyroidism should be excluded:

- *Congenital:* idiopathic GH-releasing hormone deficiency, pituitary hypoplasia, mid-facial defect and pituitary aplasia, GH gene deletion, acquired hypothalamic or pituitary tumours, cranial irradiation, head injuries, infection (meningitis encephalitis), hypothyroidism.
- *Transient:* low sex hormone concentration, psycho-social deprivation

In GH deficiency or insufficiency, the growth velocity is poor and the height less than 2SD of the mean. The bone age is delayed and the clinical appearance may be characterized by increased skin fold thickening, infantile 'doll-like facies' and micropenis.

The use of GH in these children will restore normal growth velocity after a period of catch-up growth. If the patient does not respond to the treatment, either compliance is poor or the diagnosis is incorrect.

IGF-1 levels can be helpful in the diagnosis and to assess compliance. When testing a child for GH deficiency in the prepubertal years with no signs of puberty, the child should be primed with sex steroids 2 days before the test (testosterone 100 mg for boys and ethinylestradiol 30 mg for girls).

Case 66

1. Restrictive lung disease
2. Neuromuscular disorders
   Fibrosing alveolitis

Lung function

	Obstructive	Restrictive
FVC	Low	Low
VC	Low	Low
FEV$_1$	Low	Low (proportion to FVC)
FEV$_1$/FVC	Low	Normal or high
FEF$_{25-75\%}$	Low	Low

Restrictive lung diseases

The common causes are cystic fibrosis, pulmonary infection, pulmonary oedema, fibrosing alveolitis, emphysema and neuromuscular disorders.

Obstructive lung diseases

The common causes are bronchiolitis, asthma, bronchiectasis and cystic fibrosis.

Case 67

1. Pneumothorax
   Chest illumination
2. Respiratory acidosis
3. Insert a chest drain

Respiratory acidosis

Pathophysiology

Respiratory acidosis results from inadequate pulmonary excretion of CO_2 in the presence of normal production of CO_2. CO_2 is a major component of the principal buffer system of extracellular fluid. Any rise in CO_2 should be buffered by non-bicarbonate buffers, e.g. protein, phosphate, haemoglobin, and lactate within the cell and protein in the extracellular fluid.

An increase in CO_2 and acidosis will stimulate the kidneys to increase hydrogen ion excretion as well as ammonium and titratable acid. This will lead to more bicarbonate production as well as absorption. The level of bicarbonate will increase as a result of these physiological changes. The increase in plasma bicarbonate level compensates for the primary increase of CO_2 so the pH returns towards normal and respiratory acidosis is compensated by a normal renal mechanism.

Respiratory acidosis can be due to neuromuscular disorders, airway obstruction, vascular disease, pulmonary oedema and prematurity.

Chronic lung disease of prematurity (CLDP) is mainly obstructive and leads to chronic respiratory acidosis, which can be compensated by normal renal function through the buffering mechanism.

Pneumothorax in the term newborn infant

Sudden deterioration in ventilated premature babies with gas changes and CO_2 build-up is always related to inadequate ventilation as a result of tube problems or pneumothorax.

Actions to be taken while the baby is being ventilated if oxygen require-ment is increased:

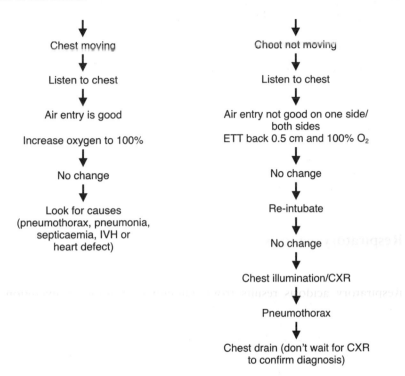

Chest moving

↓

Listen to chest

↓

Air entry is good

Increase oxygen to 100%

↓

No change

↓

Look for causes
(pneumothorax, pneumonia,
septicaemia, IVH or
heart defect)

Chest not moving

↓

Listen to chest

↓

Air entry not good on one side/
both sides
ETT back 0.5 cm and 100% O_2

↓

No change

↓

Re-intubate

↓

No change

↓

Chest illumination/CXR

↓

Pneumothorax

↓

Chest drain (don't wait for CXR
to confirm diagnosis)

Pneumothorax is estimated to occur in up to 1–2% of term infants. The commonest cause is alveolar rupture due to over-inflation. It can occur spontaneously. Symptomatic pneumothorax is characterized by respira-tory distress (increase in RR, apnoea, tachypnoea and cyanosis with grunting). Sudden deterioration is uncommon. Gradual deterioration in respiratory function is the most commonly observed scenario in term infants. Chest movement may be asymmetrical, with decreased air entry on the affected side and mediastinal shift to the opposite side if the pneu-mothorax is unilateral. Bilateral pneumothoraces are difficult to diag-nose clinically. Transillumination of the chest wall and CXR are vital diagnostic tools.

Administration of 100% oxygen can accelerate the re-absorption of free pleural air into the blood by reducing the nitrogen tension in blood. This will produce a nitrogen pressure gradient from the trapped air into the blood. The risk of oxygen toxicity should be borne in mind and weighed up against the benefit of treating the pneumothorax by giving 100% oxy-gen.

Case 68

1. Transposition of the great arteries (TGA with VSD)
2. Switch operation with VSD closure

Assessment of a newborn or child with suspected congenital heart disease

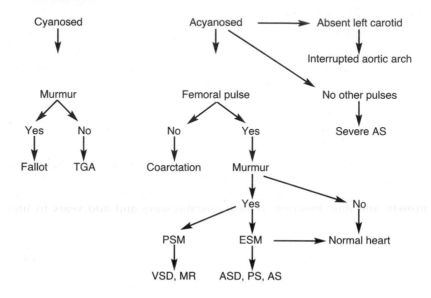

Key: AS, aortic stenosis; ASD, atrial septal defect; ESM, ejection systolic murmur; MR mitral regurgitation; PS, pulmonary stenosis; PSM pansystolic murmur; TGA, transposition of great arteries; VSD, ventricular septal defect

Transposition of the great arteries (TGA)

Saturation in the aorta is lower than that in the pulmonary artery, and is also lower than in the other chambers of the heart.

Management

- Keep the duct open by giving a prostaglandin infusion.
- Correct metabolic acidosis.
- Ventilation may be required, especially if the baby is transferred to another unit.
- Give diuretics if in cardiac failure.
- Give inotropic drugs if blood pressure is not maintained.
- Atrial septostomy can be done later by an experienced cardiologist.
- Total correction can be performed at any time, preferably early.

Case 69

1. Autosomal recessive
2. 25%
3. DNA study
   Sweat test
   Neonatal screening

Testing for cystic fibrosis (CF)

The sweat test is the most common diagnostic test for CF. At least 100 g of sweat are collected and the level of chloride measured. Chloride values between 40 and 60 mmol/l are borderline, and sweat chloride greater than 60 mmol/l is consistent with the diagnosis of CF. The cystic fibrosis transmembrane conductance regulator (*CFTR*) gene can be detected from a blood sample. Almost 800 hundred variants have been identified, the commonest of which is *F508*. *Increased faecal elastase is also evidence of possible CF.*

Neonatal screening is now available in the UK and can be very helpful in identifying cases earlier, so treatment can be started earlier and life expectancy prolonged. Early diagnosis and treatment can improve growth and lung function, reduce hospital stays and add years to life. CXR and lung function tests are helpful but not diagnostic.

If both parents are carriers, there is a 25% chance a child will have CF, a 50% chance a child will carry the CF gene but not have CF, and a 25% chance a child will not carry the gene and not have CF.

Case 70

1. Ataxia telangiectasia
2. Telangiectasia of the eyes
   Nystagmus
3. Immunoglobulins
   DNA breakage study
   Abdominal ultrasound

Ataxia telangiectasia (AT)

AT is inherited as an autosomal recessive trait associated with mutations in the *ATM* gene, and is probably due to abnormal DNA repair causing chromosomal breaks at the sites of T-cell receptor and immunoglobulin genes. AT is characterized by cerebellar ataxia with progressive neurological deterioration, oculocutaneous telangiectasia, immunodeficiency with impairment of cell-mediated immunity and antibody production, gonadal dysgenesis, chromosomal abnormalities, and malignant disorders. Alpha-fetoprotein and carcinoembryonic antigen are constant markers. Patients with AT are sensitive to irradiation, which causes cellular and chromosomal damage and may precipitate malignancy.

Investigations in acute cerebellar ataxia

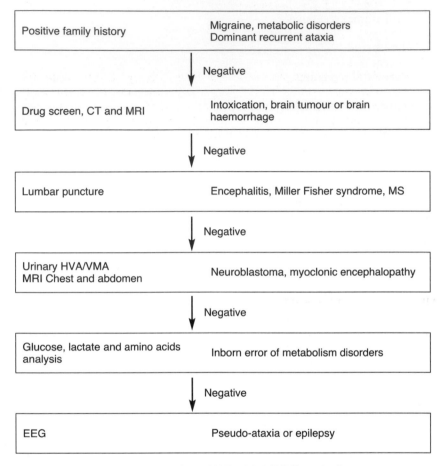

With permission from Professor Gerald M Fenichel (WB Saunders)

The figure above shows possibilities for differential diagnosis; it is not necessary for all these tests to be done. A thorough history and clinical examination is more appropriate before considering investigations.

Case 71

A 9-year-old boy presents with swelling of his face, legs and scrotum. He has been treated for iron deficiency anaemia over the last three years. He is pale, lethargic and had a distended abdomen.There is no history of diarrhoea or blood or mucus in his stool. Both parents are from Albania and there are no similar problems in the rest of the family.

Hb	8.2 g/dl
WCC	12.5×10^9/l (N 11.7, L 3.7)
Plt	460×10^9/l
U	2.4 mmol/l
Na	135 mmol/l
K	4.2 mmol/l
Cr	55 mmol/l
PT	13 s (12–14)
PTT	26.5 s (27–40)
TT	10 s (9–11)
Alb	11 mmol/l
ALK	165 mmol/l
ALT	15 mmol/l
Bilirubin	15 mmol/l
ESR	12 mm/h
CRP	15 mg/l
Urine	+ protein, no blood nor organisms
Igs	All normal
CD4:CD8 ratio	Within normal range
CXR	No abnormalities

MRI abdomen with barium and gadolinium: thickening loops of jejunum, duodenum and upper part of small intestine

1. **What is the most likely diagnosis?**
   a. CF
   b. Protein loss enteropathy
   c. Coeliac disease
   d. Inflammatory bowel disease
   e. Lymphoma

2. **What one other investigation can be done?**
   a. Upper and lower GIT biopsies
   b. Barium swallow and follow-through
   c. Abdominal ultrasound
   d. 3D abdominal CT scan
   e. White cell scan

3. **What are the first steps in managing his oedema?**
   a. Diuretics
   b. Fluid restriction
   c. Monitor urine output
   d. Albumin infusion
   e. Nasogastric feeding
   f. Monitor U&Es daily

Case 72

A 2-month-old infant presents with central cyanosis, which is not persistent. Cardiac catheterization is performed.

	O$_2$ saturation (%)	Mean pressure (mmHg)
SVC	44	
IVC	56	
RA	85	
RV	84	79
PA	84	50
PV	93	10
LA	73	
LV	84	12

1. **What is the most likely diagnosis?**
   a. VSD
   b. PDA
   c. Pulmonary stenosis
   d. Coarctation of aorta
   e. TAPVD
   f. Eisenmenger syndrome

2. **What is the most appropriate test that can be done to confirm the diagnosis?**
   a. Cardiac MRI scan
   b. Echocardiography
   c. ECG
   d. CXR
   e. Angiography

Case 73

A 2-year-old boy presents with a 7-day history of ulcerated skin lesions. No lymphadenopathy is noted. He has a history of frequent otitis media. His weight is below the 3rd centile. There are no tonsils on examination.

Hb 11 g/dl
WCC 5 × 10^9/l (N 1.0)
Plt 332 × 10^9/l
Blood culture reveals *Pseudomonas*.

1. **What are the most likely diagnoses?**

2. **Give one alternative diagnosis.**

He was treated with antibiotics. His WCC rose to 19×10^9/l with a neutrophilia. Unfortunately, he was admitted two weeks later with *Pseudomonas* osteomyelitis.

IgG   <1 g/l (6–15)
IgA   0.5 g/l (0.5–4)
IgM   0.2 g/l (0.2–4)

3.   **What is the diagnosis?**

Case 74

A child can build a tower of 8 cubes. This is what he can copy.

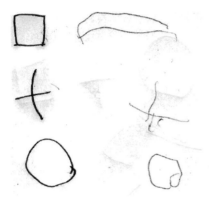 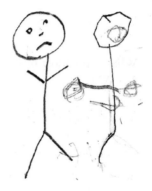

1.   **What is the nearest age you can suggest?**
    a.   18 months
    b.   2 years
    c.   30 months
    d.   36 months
    e.   42 months

2.   **How would you test his vision?**
    a.   Snellen chart
    b.   STYCAR test
    c.   White balls on black carpet
    d.   VEP
    e.   None of the above

Case 75

These are the results of CSF analysis from a 3-year-old child who was referred to Casualty by his desperate GP. He had been treated for tonsillitis with erythromycin and had become more drowsy and sleepy and had focal seizures on the right that lasted 2 minutes. There was no neck stiffness or photophobia. An EEG was also done as an emergency, and a CT scan without gadolinium showed no abnormalities.

Lumbar puncture revealed:

Pressure	18 mmHg (8–10)
WCC	30% lymphocytes
Protein	0.5 g
Glucose	3.6 mmol/l (serum glucose 5.4 mmol/l)
Gram stain	Negative

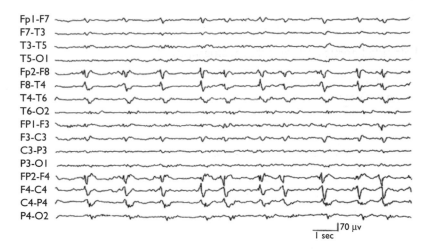

1. **What abnormalities does this EEG show?**
   a. Right periodic lateralization epileptiform discharges
   b. Generalized spike wave discharges
   c. Left periodic lateralization epileptiform discharges
   d. Periodic high-amplitude sharp and slow wave complexes
   e. None of the above

2. **What is the most likely diagnosis?**
   a. Viral meningitis
   b. Viral encephalitis
   c. Partially treated meningitis
   d. *Mycobacterium tuberculosis* meningitis
   e. Transverse myelitis

3. **What further investigations are required?**
   a. MRI brain
   b. CT brain with gadolinium
   c. PCR for HSV
   d. CXR
   e. None of the above

Case 76

These are the results of cardiac catheterization performed on a 7-month-old boy with a history of cyanosis:

Saturation   89–94% on oximetry

	Pressure
AO (D)	122/54 (85) D/S (M)
AO (arterial)	118/54 (81)
LV	121/9
LA	14/4 (9)
RA	5
RVO	97/2
RV body	112/9

Left-sided aortic arch on echocardiography

1. **What is the diagnosis?**
    a. VSD
    b. ASD
    c. Tetralogy of Fallot
    d. Transposition of the great arteries
    e. Total anomalous pulmonary venous drainage

2. **What are three risk factors at this stage?**
    a. Bacterial endocarditis
    b. Pulmonary embolism
    c. Cerebrovascular accident
    d. Cyanotic spells
    e. Heart failure
    f. Cardiac arrhythmias
    g. Pulmonary hypertension

Case 77

A 1-year-old child has a history of failure to thrive. His birthweight was 4 kg, and he has been breastfed for 6 months. At the age of one year his weight is only 8 kg.

Hb	11.2 g/dl
WCC	6.2×10^9/l
Plt	180×10^9/l
Blood film	Hypochromia, anisocytosis and acanthocytosis
X-ray of wrist shows evidence of rickets	
Serum cholesterol	0.7 mmol/l
Stool shows fat globules	

1. **What is the diagnosis and what is the mode of inheritance?**
   a. Cystic fibrosis
   b. Shwachman syndrome
   c. Ataxia telangiectasia
   d. Abetaliproteinaemia
   e. Coeliac disease

2. **How should the diagnosis be confirmed?**
   a. Upper GIT biopsy
   b. Lipid profile measurement
   c. Sweat test
   d. Endomysial antibodies
   e. Bone marrow aspiration

3. **What other clinical signs may be present?**
   a. Ataxia
   b. Retinitis pigmentosa
   c. Nystagmus
   d. Macrocephaly
   e. Short stature
   f. Tremor

Case 78

A 7-year-old child presents with status epilepticus. The seizures terminate with emergency treatment. These are the investigation results. Of note in the past is a history of pica.

Hb	7.1 g/dl
WCC	8.3×10^9/l
Plt	175×10^9/l
Ca	2.23 mmol/l
Glucose	5.2 mmol/l
Na	121 mmol/l
K	4.9 mmol/l
U	3.4 µmol/l
CSF:	
WCC	4
RBC	40
No organisms seen	
Protein	0.23 mg/l

Glc   3.1 mmol/l
Urine:
Protein   +++
Amino acid   +++

1. **What is the most likely diagnosis?**
   a. Cystinosis
   b. Tyrosinaemia
   c. Wilson disease
   d. Lead poisoning
   e. Galactosaemia

2. **List one further appropriate investigation to aid diagnosis:**
   a. Serum amino acids
   b. Serum copper and caeruloplasmin
   c. Serum lead level
   d. White cell enzymes
   e. Long bone and abdominal X-ray

Case 79

A 6-month-old infant is referred with failure to thrive. He has been constipated since birth. His milk intake is 120 ml every 2 hours. He wakes during the night crying, but he will go back to sleep after a feed of 120 ml of milk.

Na   131 mmol/l
Hb   12 g/dl
K   2.7 mmol/l
WCC 7.5×10^9/l
Cl   85 mmol/l
Plt 190×10^9/l
Cr   45 µmol/l
Protein 30 g/l
U   3.9 mmol/l
Urine:
Na   10 mmol/l
K   60 mmol/l
pH   7.50
U   200 mmol/l
HCO^{-3} 30 kPa

1. **What is the differential diagnosis?**
   a. RTA
   b. Psychogenic polydipsia
   c. Nephrogenic diabetes insipidus
   d. Diabetes mellitus
   e. Central diabetes insipidus

2. **Which investigations will aid diagnosis?**
   a. Serum osmolality
   b. Urine osmolality
   c. Renal ultrasound
   d. Water deprivation test
   e. All of the above

Case 80

A 10-year-old girl is brought to the A&E Department by her mother as she has developed worsening swelling around her eyes and ankles during the afternoon. Her father died suddenly from upper respiratory obstruction of uncertain aetiology 10 years ago.

Urine	No protein or blood
Hb	13 g/dl
WCC	8.3×10^9/l
Plt	265×10^9/l
Na	139 mmol/l
K	4.2 mmol/l
U	3.1 mmol/l
Cr	35 µmol/l
ALT	9 IU/l
ALP	12 IU/l
Bili	6 µmol/l
Alb	35 g/l
T protein	70 g/l
IgE	210 g/l
C3, C4	Normal

1. **What is the diagnosis?**
    a. Nephrotic syndrome
    b. Familial hereditary angio-oedema
    c. Acute glomerulonephritis
    d. Heart failure
    e. None of the above

2. **What is the underlying problem?**
    a. Food allergy
    b. Post-streptococcal minimal change glomerulonephritis
    c. C1 esterase inhibitor deficiency
    d. Rheumatic fever
    e. None of the above

3. **Outline your initial management of this girl:**
    a. Referral to HDU
    b. C1 esterase replacement
    c. Echocardiography
    d. Renal biopsy
    e. IV hydrocortisone and IV antihistamines

Case 71

1. Inflammatory bowel disease
2. Upper and lower GIT biopsies
3. Monitor urine output
    Monitor U&E daily

Crohn disease

Crohn disease is an idiopathic, chronic, transmural inflammatory process. It can affect the entire GIT system from mouth to anus, often leading to fibrosis and obstructive symptoms. No cause has been identified, but there are many theories that it may be caused by genetic, microbial, immunological, environmental, dietary, vascular and even psychosocial factors. The initial presentation may be with loss of weight, diarrhoea and short stature, or abdominal pain with the suggestion of intestinal obstruction. It may present with anal fissure or fistulae or abscess. Patients may also present with episcleritis, uveitis, erythema nodosum and pyoderma gangrenosum, or peripheral arthritis.

Anaemia (folate, B_{12} or iron deficiency anaemia), high white cell and platelet counts, and high CRP and ESR are associated with inflammatory bowel diseases. Hypoalbuminaemia, hypercholesterolaemia, hypocalcaemia, hypomagnesaemia and hypoprothrombinaemia may reflect malabsorption. Other tests that may help to differentiate between ulcerative colitis and Crohn's disease are p-ANCA antigen (a myeloperoxidase antigen) and ASCA (anti-*S. cerevisiae* antibodies). Positive p-ANCA antigen and negative ASCA suggest the diagnosis of ulcerative colitis; conversely, positive ASCA and negative p-ANCA antigen suggest the presence of Crohn's disease.

Barium swallow and enema may show a cobblestone appearance, fistulae or strictures. MRI scan with contrast may show the same, together with thickened bowel loops, and is more specific than barium swallow or enema. The diagnostic test is upper and lower GIT endoscopy, which will show transmural involvement with non-caseating granulomas in about 50% of cases as well as patchy skip lesions. Lymphoid aggregates may also be seen throughout the bowel wall.

Algorithm for the diagnosis of chronic diarrhoea

Stool culture and reducing substances, immunoglobulins, RAST test	Infection, tropical sprue, protein intolerance disaccharidase deficiency

↓ Negative

Abdominal ultrasound and abdominal X-ray Sweat test, IRT, DNA linkage study (Δ508)	Chronic constipation, toddler's diarrhoea, cystic fibrosis Pancreatic enzyme deficiency

↓ Negative

Low platelets, neutropenia, skeletal abnormalities, pancreatic enzyme deficiency	Shwachman syndrome

↓ Negative

Conjugated hyperbilirubinaemia, abnormal LFT and clotting, abdominal ultrasound	Biliary atresia

↓ Negative

Small and large intestine biopsy, immunoglobulin levels	IBD, coeliac disease, immune deficiency

Case 72

1. Total anomalous pulmonary venous drainage with ASD (TAPVD + ASD)
2. ECG

Total anomalous pulmonary venous drainage

The saturation in the RA and RV is higher than that on the left side of the heart, which suggests that the pulmonary veins join the systemic venous system before entering the right atrium. The pulmonary artery pressure is high, as pulmonary hypertension is commonly associated with TAPVD. The prognosis is poor unless surgery is performed early.

The pulmonary veins may enter the RA, SVC or IVC, ductus venosum, or hepatic veins. The condition is usually associated with an ASD and can be divided into supra- or infra-diaphragmatic according to the entry of the pulmonary veins into the venous system. In the newborn, it usually presents with intermittent cyanosis, tachypnoea and a systolic murmur. In cases where there is severe obstruction of the pulmonary venous return, the baby will present with cyanosis and no murmurs. If there is a left-to-right shunt at the atrial or ventricular level, patients usually present with congestive cardiac failure in early life and pulmonary hypertension. ECG will show RV hypertrophy (V4R, V1) and a tall spiked P wave. CXR will show the characteristic 'snowman' or 'figure of eight' shape.

Case 73

1. X-linked hypogammaglobulinaemia
   Leukocyte adhesion deficiency (LAD)
   Chronic granulomatous disease (CGD)
2. Severe combined immune deficiency syndrome (SCID)
3. X-linked hypogammaglobulinaemia

Immunological disorders may affect children in early life.

Disease	Clinical criteria	Functional defect	Pathogenesis	Inheritance
Leukocyte adhesion deficiency (LAD)	Delayed separation of umbilical cord Skin infection and gingivitis Deep abscess and osteomyelitis	Decrease in phagocytosis and adherence	Absence of adhesion CD11a,b,c due to defect in CD118 on neutrophils, lymphocytes	AR
Chronic granulomatous disease (CGD)	Repeated infection with catalase-negative bacteria Granuloma formation	Decreased oxidative metabolism, decreased microbiocidal activity	Lack of cytochromes	X-linked recessive, AR
X-linked hypogamma-globulinaemia	Repeated bacterial infection	Panhypogamma-globulinaemia Reduced antibody activity Isohaemagglutinin not detected Lymphocyte function normal	B cells absent T cells normal	X-linked recessive

Case 74

1. 36 months
2. STYCAR test

Visual assessment in different age groups

- Ask the parents about any problems with vision in the child.
- Eye examination with examination of the fundus in all age groups.
- In neonates and younger infants, observe the child to see if he/she can fix on and follow an object or human face at a distance of 3 metres.
- Below 2½ years, use 10 white balls of varying sizes (from one-eighth to 2½ inches in diameter) that are rolled on a dark strip horizontally to the line of the infant's gaze, some 3 metres from the child. It is important to note that visualization of even the smallest ball does not mean that the vision is perfect.

- The STYCAR (Sheridan) letter test can be started from 2½ years of age by matching letters as follows. Present a single letter of decreasing size at 3 metres. The child has a key card that has five (2½–3½ years), seven (3½–4½ years) or nine (5–7 years) capital letters on it.
- The Key Picture Test is similar to the STYCAR letter test but uses pictures and can be used by some children as young as 18 months.
- Snellen charts can be used from the age of 7 years.
- Visual evoked response (VER) to flashes is an excellent technique to demonstrate the integrity of the visual pathways without patient cooperation. By the age of 3 months, the morphology and latency of the VER are relatively mature, but interpretation may still be difficult.

Case 75

1. Right periodic lateralization epileptiform discharges
2. Viral encephalitis
3. PCR for HSV from CSF
   MRI brain or CT scan

Herpes simplex encephalitis

Herpes simplex infections are asymptomatic in 80% of patients. There are two types: type 1 (HSV-1) and type 2 (HSV-2). HSV-2 more commonly causes encephalitis in newborns and infants, whereas HSV-1 is more common in adult encephalitis. The two are closely related but differ in epidemiology. HSV-1 is transmitted chiefly by contact with infected saliva, whereas HSV-2 is transmitted sexually or from a mother's genital tract infection to her newborn. The virus remains latent and is reactivated when the patient becomes febrile, or is exposed to emotional stress, trauma or sunlight, and during menstruation. The trigeminal ganglia are involved most commonly with HSV-1 and the sacral nerve root ganglia (S2–S5) are involved with HSV-2 infection.

Approximately 80% of children with HSV encephalitis do not have a history of labial herpes. They may present with neurological deficits, seizures, delirium, lethargy, confusion and coma. There may also be meningeal signs and headache. The CT scan shows areas of low-density attenuation at the temporal lobes in about two-thirds of patients in the first 3–4 days after presentation. It may show some enhancement. MRI is more sensitive and may show changes even earlier than 3 days after the initial presentation. It may show haemorrhagic lesions in the temporal lobes. EEG will show focal temporal changes, or diffuse slowing may be observed. Lumbar puncture will show mildly elevated protein, normal glucose and a moderate pleocytosis (mostly mononuclear cells). PCR for HSV is very sensitive and 80% specific.

Treatment includes IV aciclovir for 3 weeks and oral aciclovir for 3 weeks. Follow-up is recommended on a regular basis for the first year; if there are no epileptic seizures and the child is developmentally intact, he/she can be discharged.

Case 76

1. Tetralogy of Fallot
2. Cyanotic spells
   Pulmonary embolism
   Bacterial endocarditis

Tetralogy of Fallot (ToF)

Cardiac catheterization and angiography are still performed before or during surgery to provide more information. The ECG in ToF will show right ventricular hypertrophy and right axis deviation. Echocardiography is the diagnostic procedure, with evaluation of pulmonary artery pressure. Approximately 20–30% of patients with ToF will show a right aortic arch. Chest X-ray will show oligaemic lung.

Treatment is divided into palliative surgery and total correction. Palliative surgery (Blalock–Taussig shunt) can be done after birth if the infant presents with severe ToF. Total correction is usually done after the first year of life, depending on the size of the child and the symptoms.

Treatment of cyanotic spells:

- 100% oxygen via facial mask.
- IV propranolol and then maintenance.
- Watch for side effects in asthmatics, and may cause low blood sugar.
- Correct metabolic acidosis with colloids or bicarbonate.
- Check haematocrit, haemoglobin and clotting.

Case 77

1. Abetalipoproteinaemia (AR)
2. Lipid profile measurement
3. Ataxia and retinitis pigmentosa

Abetalipoproteinaemia

Clinical features

Abetalipoproteinaemia is an autosomal recessive disorder resulting from lack of synthesis of apoprotein B, which is essential for the formation of low-density lipoprotein (LDL), very low-density lipoprotein (VLDL) and chylomicrons. Homozygotes will have no chylomicrons, LDL or VLDL. The cholesterol level is <1.3 mmol/l and triglycerides are <0.2 mmol/l. Heterozygotes have no clinical or biochemical abnormality.

The patient presents with features of fat malabsorption and diarrhoea. Bleeding may occur due to vitamin K malabsorption, and there may be signs and symptoms of malabsorption of other fat-soluble vitamins. Acanthocytosis (spiky red cells) is always present from birth, but is not pathognomonic.

Diagnosis

The diagnosis can be confirmed by lipid electrophoresis, which will show absence of LDL.

Evoked retinography (ERG) is extinguished, the serum cholesterol level is low, EMG shows denervation and conduction velocities are diminished.

Management and prognosis

Retinitis pigmentosa and ataxia appear by the end of the first decade and are gradually progressive. The neurological features are partly due to prolonged vitamin E deficiency. Cardiac arrhythmias can occur and may lead to sudden death. Treatment with vitamin E prevents the development of or progression of eye and nervous diseases (Havel and Kane 2001). Vitamins K, A and D and a low-fat diet are also recommended. Medium-chain fatty acids can be used as a substitute for other fatty acids.

Case 78

1. Lead encephalopathy
2. Serum lead level
   Long bone and abdominal X-ray

Lead poisoning

Pathophysiology

Lead toxicity leads to disturbance of porphyrin synthesis and coproporphyrinuria. It also interferes with the breakdown of RNA by inhibiting pyrimidine 5-nucleotidase, causing the appearance of punctate basophilia. There are also disturbances in carbohydrate metabolism, cell membrane transport and renal tubular absorption. The toxic level at which signs and symptoms may appear varies from child to child. Symptoms are unlikely if the whole blood lead level is <2.5 µmol/l. Some behavioural problems and learning difficulties can manifest with a lead level between 1.4 and 2.9 µmol/l. Sources of lead poisoning vary from sucking or chewing lead paint to an Indian makeup for the eyes that contains high levels of lead.

Clinical features

Chronic lead poisoning may present with abdominal pain, pallor, anorexia, irritability and failure to thrive. In the acute stage, drowsiness, convulsion and coma may be the initial presentation (encephalopathic picture). Some children can present with intellectual impairment alone. Hypochromic, microcytic anaemia is common with punctate basophilia.

There is increased urinary coproporphyrin and laevulinic acid. On X-ray, increased bone density with transverse bands at the end of long bones is seen.

Management

The first measure to be taken is removal of the source of lead poisoning. D-Penicillinamine is given in mild cases, 910 mg/kg orally twice a day. In severe poisoning, sodium calcium edetate (EDTA), 40 mg/kg IV infusion over 1 hour twice a day for 5 days, or deep muscle injection of dimercaprol should be given.

Case 79

1. Psychogenic polydipsia
    Nephrogenic diabetes insipidus
    Central diabetes insipidus
2. All of the above

Anion gap = Na − (Cl + HCO^{-3})

Normal anion gap (10–14) and hyperchloraemia	Increased anion gap (>14) and normochloraemia
Diarrhoea, fistula	Increased acid load
Proximal renal tubular acidosis	Organic acidaemia
Distal renal tubular acidosis	Lactic acidosis (primary or secondary)
Drugs (carbonic anhydrase inhibitor)	Ketoacidosis

Other causes of hypokalaemia:

• Pyloric stenosis with low plasma Cl, K and positive feeding test.
• Chloride syndrome with generalized aminoaciduria, RTA and normal Cl level.
• Primary and secondary hyperaldosteronism associated with high blood pressure.
• Distal RTA with urine pH of >6.

Case 80

1. Familial hereditary angio-oedema
2. C1 esterase inhibitor deficiency
3. IV hydrocortisone and IV antihistamines
    Referral to HDU

Familial hereditary angio-oedema

The condition is inherited as an autosomal dominant trait and develops late in childhood. There is a deficiency of protein control of C1 esterase inhibitor, which leads to localized oedema without urticaria. The oedema occurs spontaneously anywhere in the body. It may cause upper airway obstruction, which is life-threatening. Patients may present with abdominal pain and can be misdiagnosed as having a surgical problem.

The C4 is persistently low even between attacks; this is mainly due to massive consumption of this factor. C1NH level is variable (very low circulating protein or the protein is functionally defective in 15% of patients). Management in acute presentations may include fresh frozen plasma after initial resuscitation.

Danazol is the treatment of choice and raises functional C1 esterase inhibitor level sufficiently to prevent attacks. Contraceptive preparations may help in girls in the post-pubertal period.

Case 81

A 2-month-old infant presents to the A&E Department with a recent onset of lethargy and irritability. She has been breastfed normally, although she received mixed fruit juice on the day of admission, when she was staying with a family friend. She is vomiting intermittently on admission. Investigations reveal:

Blood glucose   1.3 mmol/l
pH   7.2 kPa
HCO^{-3} 12 kPa
U   4.6 mmol/l
Cr   28 µmol/l
Lactate   6.2 mmol/l
Urine   Glycosuria, aminoaciduria and proteinurea
Non-glucose reducing substances in urine by Clinitest

1. **What is the probable diagnosis?**
    a. UTI
    b. Inborn error of metabolism
    c. Pyloric stenosis
    d. Hypothyroidism
    e. Nesidioblastosis

2. **How would you confirm the diagnosis?**
    a. Serum amino acids
    b. MSU
    c. Abdominal ultrasound
    d. Thyroid function test
    e. Liver biopsy

Case 82

A 2-year-old girl is referred with poor weight gain and a history of intermittent vomiting. There is no history of diarrhoea or abdominal pain. Abdominal US, CXR and barium swallow are normal.

pH study excludes gastro-oesophageal reflux.

Urine – no growth of three specimens.

Na   137 mmol/l
K   4.3 mmol/l
Cl   118 mmol/l
U   3.9 mmol/l
Cr   41 µmol/l
HCO^{-3} 10 mmol/l
pH   7.19
Urine   pH 5.1, no aminoaciduria or glycosuria

1. **What is the diagnosis?**
    a. UTI
    b. Food intolerance
    c. Proximal renal tubular acidosis
    d. Distal renal tubular acidosis
    e. Nephrogenic diabetes insipidus

2. **How can your diagnosis be confirmed?**
    a. Ammonium chloride loading test
    b. DMSA scan
    c. Barium swallow
    d. Water deprivation test
    e. MSU

3. **List four aetiological causes.**
    a. Galactosaemia
    b. Wilson disease
    c. Heavy metal poisoning
    d. Glycogen storage diseases
    e. Fructosuria
    f. Haemosiderosis
    g. Cystinosis
    h. Cystinuria

Case 83

A 2-year-old boy is seen in clinic with a history of persistent systolic murmur. He has suffered repeated chest infections, but his parent-held record showed a reasonable pattern of growth and development. Cardiac catheterization is performed.

	Pressure (mmHg)	O₂ saturation (%)
RA	5	68
RV		66
PA	33/15 (24)	80
LA	5	96
LV	95/42	95
AO	95/40 (62)	95

1. What is the diagnosis?

2. How would you treat this condition?

3. What are the possible treatment modalities available in the neonatal period?

Case 84

An 11-year-old girl is seen in the Chest Clinic with a history of chronic cough and poor growth development. Lung function tests are performed:

	Pre-salbutamol	Post-salbutamol	Normal values
FVC (ml)	1900	2200	(1950–3400)
FEV_1 (ml)	1650	2100	(1620–2915)
TLC (ml)	2600	2700	(2700–2900)
FEV_1/FVC (%)	87	95	

1. **What is the most likely diagnosis?**
   a. Fibrosing alveolitis
   b. Pulmonary infection
   c. Obstructive lung disease
   d. Cystic fibrosis
   e. Neuromuscular disorders

2. **What further tests can be done to help in managing her condition?**
   a. Sputum culture
   b. Immunoglobulin levels
   c. Bronchoscopy
   d. Ciliary function
   e. Sweat test

Case 85

A 10-year-old boy presents with hepatomegaly measuring 2 cm and abdominal pain. The blood is described by the laboratory technician as 'turbid plasma'. The boy's father died at the age of 45 years following a heart attack due to coronary heart disease.

Na	124 mmol/l
K	3.0 mmol/l
U	4.1 mmol/l
Cr	24 µmol/l
Glucose	4 mmol/l
Amylase	1100 mmol/l

1. **What investigation should be done to help in diagnosis?**
   a. Echocardiography
   b. Abdominal ultrasound
   c. Fasting lipid profile
   d. Blood film
   e. Liver biopsy

2. **What is the most likely diagnosis?**

Case 86

These are the results of cardiac catheterization of a 36-hour-old infant with a history of cyanosis and no other abnormality on systemic examination. A full septic screen was subsequently negative.

	Pressure (mmHg)	O₂ saturation (%)
SVC	10	55
IVC	10	72
RA	9	60
RV	80/8	60
LA	3	65
LV	90/7	62
AO		64

1. What is the diagnosis?
2. How may the diagnosis be confirmed?
3. What is your immediate management of this infant prior to surgery?

Case 87

A 4-year-old boy is referred. He can walk but not run. He often trips over. He can copy a circle, cross and square. He knows six colours and occasionally speaks three-word sentences. He can understand game rules and shares them with others.

1. What is the differential diagnosis?
2. What is his gross motor development age?
3. List three investigations that might aid diagnosis.

Case 88

This is the composition of milk per 100 ml used by a mother for her 9-month-old daughter:

Protein 1.56 g/l
Fat   3.6 g/l
Na   0.78 mmol
K   1.67 mmol
PO₄   0.87 mmol/l
Ca   1.11 mmol
CHO   7.3 g/l

1. What type of milk is this?
2. What is the difference between this milk and breast milk?

Case 89

A 4-year-old boy presents with epistaxis. Both parents are Greek Cypriots by birth. There is no haemarthrosis and no family history of a similar problem. Haematological investigations reveals:

PTT   110 s (40)
TT   2 min (7)
PT   13 s (14)
Plt   110 × 10⁹/l
WCC   4.2 × 10⁹/l (normal differential)
Hb   9 g/dl
Ret   60%

1. **What is the diagnosis?**
    a.   Haemophilia A
    b.   Von Willebrand disease
    c.   Vitamin K deficiency
    d.   Haemophilia B
    e.   None of the above

2. **What is the emergency treatment for this condition?**
    a.   IM vitamin K
    b.   Fresh frozen plasma
    c.   Factor VIII replacement
    d.   Fresh blood
    e.   Factor XI replacement

Case 90

A 5-year-old girl is admitted with a history of drowsiness and unsteady gait. She suffered a generalized tonic-clonic seizure at home. She had similar episodes at the age of 8 months and 16 months. Her sibling died at the age of 6 months with progressive seizure disorder and failure to thrive. Investigation reveals:

Na   140 mmol/l
K   4.00 mmol/l
U   3.4 µmol/l
Cr   28 mmol/l
Glucose   5.0 mmol/l
Lactate   1.7 mmol/l
LFT   Normal
Ammonia   600 µmol/l (80 mmol/l)
Anion gap   <20
Ketones   Low
CSF:
WCC   1
RBC   <3
Glucose   3.1
Lactate   <1
Protein   34 mg/l

Pressure 9 cmH$_2$O
EEG Generalized slow spike waves

1. **What is the most likely diagnosis?**
    a. Propionic aciduria
    b. Glutaric aciduria
    c. Urea cycle defect
    d. Ketotic hyperglycinaemia
    e. Very long-chain acyl CoA dehydrogenase deficiency (LCAD)

2. **What further testing can be carried out?**
    a. Liver biopsy
    b. Cranial MRI scan
    c. CSF glycine/pyruvate ratio
    d. Serum amino acids
    e. Skin biopsy for tissue fibroblasts

Case 81

1. Inborn error of metabolism (fructose intolerance: fructose-1,6-diphosphatase deficiency or fructose-1-phosphate aldolase deficiency)
2. Liver biopsy

Fructose intolerance

The history of lethargy, irritability, sweating and drowsiness is suggestive of hypoglycaemia which could be secondary to a metabolic illness. This does not happen while the baby is on breastmilk. In this case, the child has had for the first time a fruit juice, which is rich in fructose.

Fructose 1-phosphate aldolase deficiency

This is also called hereditary fructose intolerance or fructosaemia. There is a deficiency of the enzyme fructose-1,6-bisphosphate aldolase B. Children may present with vomiting, hypoglycaemia, failure to thrive, cachexia, hepatomegaly, jaundice, coagulopathy, severe metabolic acidosis, lactic acidosis, coma, renal Fanconi syndrome, hyperuricaemia, lactic acidaemia, proximal tubular acidosis, aminoaciduria, glycosuria, phosphaturia or renal tubular acidosis. The diagnosis may be suspected by the presence of non-glucose reducing sugar, elimination of fructose and dietary history. Liver biopsy is the diagnostic test for any of the above enzyme deficiencies. The fructose tolerance test should be done with IV fructose, not oral, as the latter may cause violent gastrointestinal symptoms.

Fructose intolerance is manifested in three inherited metabolic disorders:

	Fructokinase deficiency	Fructose-1,6-diphosphatase deficiency Fructose-1,6-bisphosphate aldolase B deficiency
Inheritance	AR	AR (more common)
Pathophysiology	Blockage of fructose metabolism in liver, kidney, intestine but not in muscle and adipose tissues	Gluconeogenesis impairment in both
Presentation	No symptoms	Late after introduction of fruits in both
		Hypoglycaemia is the most common presentation
		Hepatosplenomegaly

Investigations	Fructosuria	Fructosuria, hypoglycaemia, Fanconi syndrome-like picture, lactic acidosis
		Fructose-1,6-bisphophate aldolase B deficiency in white cells or enzymes and fibroblasts. Liver biopsy may be required in fructose-1,6-diphosphatase deficiency, as the enzyme is difficult to detect in fibroblasts
Management	Probably nothing Counselling	Genetic counselling and prenatal diagnosis is possible
		Treatment of acute presentation
		Life-long fructose-free diet
		Liver transplant?

Case 82

1. Proximal (primary) renal tubular acidosis
2. Ammonium chloride loading test
3. Galactosaemia; Wilson disease; heavy metal poisoning, e.g. lead, mercury; glycogen storage diseases

Renal tubular acidosis (RTA)

	Distal renal tubular acidosis	Proximal renal tubular acidosis
Proteinuria	No	Yes
Glycosuria	No	Yes
Phosphaturia	No	Yes
Bicarbonaturia	No	Yes
Urine pH	Alkaline	If HCO^{-3} >16–18 mmol/l, pH >5.5 If HCO^{-3} <16–18 mmol/l, pH <5.5
Calcium	Increased	Increased
Plasma chloride	Increased	Increased
HCO^{-3}	Low	Low
K	Low	Low
Nephrocalcinosis	Yes	No?
Inheritance	AD/X-linked and sporadic	AR/AD/X-linked and sporadic
Treatment	$NaHCO_3$ (2–5 mmol/kg/day), K, HCO^{-3}/or citrate if K low	$NaHCO_3$, K, correct acidosis Vitamin D (treat the cause)

Case 83

1. Patent ductus arteriosus
2. Ligation or transvenous umbrella ablation
3. Fluid restriction
   Indometacin

Patent ductus arteriosus (PDA)

Causes

PDA is commonly associated with maternal rubella infection during early pregnancy. It is also common in premature babies. PDA that persists beyond the first few weeks of life will rarely close spontaneously. In premature babies, if early surgical ligation or pharmacological closure of PDA is not required, spontaneous closure will occur in most of the babies.

Pathophysiology

If the PDA is small then the pressure in the right ventricle and atrium as well as the pulmonary artery is normal. If the PDA is large, pulmonary artery pressure will elevate to the systemic level and may lead to a high risk of developing pulmonary vascular disease. Also, a large PDA may cause congestive cardiac failure.

Clinical features

There will be a wide pulse pressure and a bounding pulse. The murmur is a machinery murmur heard on the chest in the second intercostal space and on interscapular auscultation. A thrill is common, and the heart size is normal on chest X-ray. The ECG will show biventricular hypertrophy. On echocardiography, the left atrium/aortic ratio is increased and the left atrium/left ventricular dimension is also increased.

A continuous murmur may be heard with the following conditions:

- Aorto-pulmonary window defect
- Sinus of Valsalva aneurysm
- Coronary arterio-venous fistulae
- Pulmonary artery branch stenosis
- Peripheral arterio-venous fistulae
- VSD and aortic valve incompetence
- Aortic valve incompetence and mitral incompetence in rheumatic fever.

Management

There is a risk of heart failure and subacute bacterial endocarditis at any age. Pulmonary hypertension is not a contraindication for closure at any age if, at catheterization, the flow is still predominantly left to right and there is no severe pulmonary vascular disease. New closure techniques besides transvenous umbrella ligation include thoracoscopic surgical ligation; this technique is used in large centres.

Case 84

1. Obstructive lung disease
2. Sweat test
   Immunoglobulin levels
   Bronchoscopy and biliary function

Restrictive lung disease

The common causes are cystic fibrosis, pulmonary infection, pulmonary oedema, fibrosing alveolitis and neuromuscular disorders.

Obstructive lung disease

The common causes are bronchiolitis, asthma, bronchiectasis and cystic fibrosis.

Lung function

Spirometry is the first lung function test done. It measures how much and how quickly air can move out of lungs. For this test, the patient breathes into a mouthpiece attached to a recording device (spirometer). The information collected by the spirometer may be printed out on a chart called a spirogram.

The more common lung function values measured with spirometry are:

- **Forced vital capacity (FVC)** is the maximum volume of gas that can be expired as forcefully and rapidly as possible after a maximum inspiration. This can be measured in litres per minute by a spirometer. FVC is normally equal to a slow vital capacity (VC). FVC and VC should be within 5% of each other. In obstructive lung disease the FVC is lower than the VC.
- **Forced expiratory volume in 1 second (FEV$_1$)** is the volume of gas expired in the first second from the beginning of FVC measurement. It is reduced in obstructive lung disease whether it involves small or large airways. In restrictive lung diseases, e.g. cystic fibrosis, fibrosing alveolitis, etc., it is also reduced but remains proportional to FVC. This is not the case in obstructive lung disease, in which FVC is preserved and FEV$_1$ value is reduced.
- **FEV$_1$/FVC ratio** is reduced in obstructive lung disease and is normal or high in restrictive lung disease.
- **Forced expiration flow 25–75% (FEF$_{25-75\%}$)** is the average flow during the middle volume of the FVC manoeuvre. The FEF$_{25-75\%}$ may suggest changes in the small airways and should not be used to diagnose the defects in small airways. It is reduced in both restrictive and obstructive lung disease.

Peak expiratory flow (PEF). This measures how quickly the patient can exhale. It is usually measured at the same time as FVC.

Maximum voluntary ventilation (MVV). This measures the greatest amount of air the patient can breathe in and out during one minute.

Slow vital capacity (SVC). This measures the amount of air the patient can slowly exhale after inhaling as deeply as possible.

Total lung capacity (TLC). This measures the amount of air in a patient's lungs after he/she has inhaled as deeply as possible.

Functional residual capacity (FRC). This measures the amount of air in the patient's lungs at the end of a normal exhaled breath.

Expiratory reserve volume (ERV). This measures the difference between the amount of air in a patient's lungs after a normal exhale (FRC) and the amount after the patient has exhaled with force (RV).

Case 85

1. Fasting lipid profile
2. Familial hyperchylomicronaemia

Familial hyperchylomicronaemia (lipoprotein lipase deficiency)

The history of hepatomegaly and turbid plasma indicates a defect in lipid metabolism. This is an autosomal recessive disorder due to protein lipase deficiency; it is characterized by eruptive xanthomata, and abdominal pain occurring later during childhood. It sometimes presents with hepatosplenomegaly and lipaemia reticularis in asymptomatic patients. The plasma is turbid. Triglyceride is high and the cholesterol level is also high (3–10 mg/dl). Abdominal pain is an indication of pancreatitis. Medium-chain fatty acid (MCT) can be used instead of other fats in the food of these patients. The fat requirement should be 2–3 g/24 h.

Case 86

1. Total anomalous pulmonary venous drainage (TAPVD)
2. Echocardiography or MRI
3. Prostaglandin infusion
   Correct acidosis
   Oxygen
   Give diuretics if in heart failure
   Refer for atrial septostomy and cardiac repair

TAPVD (infra-diaphragmatic)

All blood returns to the RA in this condition. The pulmonary venous blood may enter the RA, SVC, IVC or ductus venosus. The condition is usually associated with ASD.

During the neonatal period and in severe obstruction of pulmonary venous return, the infant may present with intermittent cyanosis, tachypnoea and no murmurs. Another group can present with congestive heart failure in early life. There will be a large left-to-right shunt and pulmonary hypertension; the child is usually ill. ECG shows right ventricular hypertrophy with a tall R wave in V_{4R} and V_1 and a spiked tall P wave in all leads. Chest X-ray will show a 'cottage loaf' or 'figure 8' appearance of the heart. The diagnosis can be made by echocardiography. Cardiac catheterization can be done prior to surgery, or at the time of surgery. This will show that oxygen saturation is equal in RA, RV, LA and LV, and higher in venous blood before entering the heart.

Pulmonary hypertension is common during infancy and, without surgery, the prognosis is poor. Acute presentation at birth is an indication to keep the duct open until further surgery is performed or atrial septostomy carried out if the duct is closed.

Case 87

1. Myopathies
   Cerebral palsy
2. 12–15 months
3. Creatine kinase (CK)
   Electromyography (EMG)
   Brain and muscle MRI

Myopathies

The symptoms of myopathies can be classified as:

- Abnormal gait (toe-walking, waddling, ataxic)
- Easy fatigability
- Frequent falls
- Slow motor development
- Specific disability with hand grip, climbing stairs, arm elevation and rising from the floor

The myopathies are characterized by depressed tendon reflexes (not in all myopathies), raised CK, normal nerve conduction study and brief, small-amplitude polyphasic motor units on EMG. The muscle biopsy in myopathies is characterized by fibre necrosis, fatty replacement and excessive collagen. The clinical signs of myopathies can be atrophy or hypertrophy, fasciculations, joint contracture, myotonia and weakness.

	Inheritance	CK	EMG	Muscle biopsy
Neuropathy	AR/AD	N/H	Fasciculation, denervation	Group atrophy
Myopathy	AR/AD	H	Brief, small-amplitude polyphasic motor units	Group typing fibre necrosis, fatty and excessive collagen
Myasthenia	AR	N	N	Normal excessive collagen
Inflammatory myopathies	–	N	Fibrillation sharp waves at rest, polyphasic potentials	Perifascicular atrophy
Metabolic myopathies	AR	N	Non-specific	Specific enzyme
Endocrine myopathies	AR/AD	N	Non-specific	Non-specific

N, normal; H, high

With permission from Jean Aicardi (MacKeith Press)

Case 88

1. Cow & Gate Premium
2. High protein, calcium and phosphorus

Breast and formula feeding

Weaning can be initiated at 4–6 months of age, but then there are problems of potentiating allergies and causing a deficiency of trace elements, iron and vitamins.

The food for first-stage weaning should contain no added sugar or salt; it should be fairly bland in taste and very smooth in consistency, e.g. pureed fruits and vegetables.

Cows' milk can be introduced by the age of one year, as the risk of allergy and iron deficiency will be less. Healthy eating should be introduced as early as 5 years of age.

The role of vitamin K in haemorrhagic disease of the newborn in breast-fed babies remains unclear. Vitamin K is significantly high in colostrum. The oral supplementation of vitamin K in both baby and mother has a beneficial effect on vitamin K levels in babies in the early days of life.

Various types of milk that can be used in children

Type of milk	Description	Age of introduction	Use
Nutramigen Pregestimil Pepti-Junior	Protein hydrolysate	Any time after weaning	Whole protein intolerance Milk/lactose intolerance Food allergy
Calogen (LCT) Liquigen (MCT)	Liquid fat emulsion	At any age when needed	Toddler diarrhoea High-calorie diet Slowing gastric emptying
Semi-elemental: Nutramigen Pregestimil Pepti-Junior Peptid 0–2	Elemental-based formula	At any age when needed	Malabsorption states Severe food allergy/ intolerance
Elemental: Neocate Neocate Advance	Elemental-based formula	At any age when needed	Inflammatory bowel disease Protracted diarrhoea
Duocal	Soluble mix fat/carbohydrate	At any age when needed	Failure to thrive
Paediasure Nutriprem II	Whey-based high-fat/protein formula	At any age when needed	Failure to thrive Children on limited intake
Prejomin	Protein hydrolysate	At any age when needed	Infant with cystic fibrosis

Case 89

1. Haemophilia A or B
2. Factor VIII for type A and fresh frozen plasma for type B

	Haemophilia A	Haemophilia B
Inheritance factors	X-linked recessive	X-linked recessive
	Factor VIII	Factor IX
	75% reduction in activity and antigen	25% reduction in activity and normal antigen
Severity	<1% (1 unit/dl) of normal activity (severe)	Factor IX reduction will have same severity as haemophilia A
	1–5% (moderate)	
	6–30% (mild)	
Crossing placenta	No	No
Haemarthrosis	Yes	No
PTT	Prolonged	Prolonged
PT	Normal	Normal
BT	Normal	Normal
Platelets	Normal	Normal
Treatment	25–50 units of factor VIII will raise factor VIII in the recipient to 50–100% (cryoprecipitate)	Fresh frozen plasma Infusion of 100 units/kg of factor IX is required to raise factor IX to 100%
	10–15% will develop factor VIII inhibitor. It is essential to continue to give factor VIII in these patients; plasmapheresis is helpful in high levels Immunosuppressive drugs have no value	

Case 90

1. Urea cycle disorder
2. Liver biopsy

Urea cycle disorder (UCD)

Patients with a UCD can present at any time from birth to adulthood with symptoms depending on the degree of the enzyme defect. The hallmark of this condition is hyperammonaemia. A definitive diagnosis can be obtained with enzyme assays.

Hyperammonaemia is responsible for encephalopathy in these patients. It causes swelling of the astrocytes, leading to cerebral oedema and alteration of cerebral blood flow. All of these factors can cause the neurological manifestations in UCD.

Clinical features

Anorexia, vomiting and sleep disturbances in long-standing hyperammonaemia may be due to increased brain uptake of tryptophan and thus increased brain serotonin turnover. The latter may be produced by benzoate, which is used in treatment. The majority of patients present with symptoms during the neonatal period.

Treatment

In the acute form, urgent removal of nitrogen waste products is required. Kidney dialysis with supportive treatment is needed. Later, high protein intake should be avoided and benzoate and phenyl acetate used for ammonia disposal. Liver transplantation may be the only therapeutic option available for patients with recurrent acute exacerbations of UCD.

Differential diagnosis of causes of hyperammonaemia (Aicardi 1998)

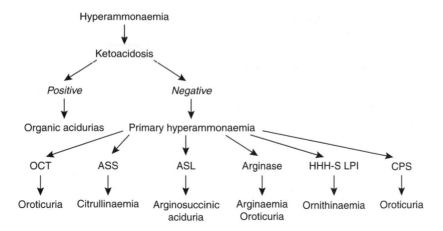

Key. OCT, ornithine transcarbamylase; ASS, arginine succinate synthetase; ASL, arginosuccinate lyase; HHH-S, hyperammonaemia, hyperornithinaemia, homocitrullinuria syndrome; LPI, lysinuric protein intolerance; CPS, carbamyl phosphate synthetase.

With permission from Jean Aicardi (MacKeith Press)

Case 91

A full-term baby is delivered vaginally with a birthweight of 3.750 kg. He is markedly pale and does not feed well. His septic screen is negative. Clotting is normal, as are LFT, blood gas and lactate.

Hb   9.2 g/dl
WCC $15 \times 10^9/l$
Plt $166 \times 10^9/l$
CRP   <5 mg/l

1. **What is the most likely diagnosis?**
   a. ABO incompatibility
   b. Congenital heart disease
   c. Inborn error of metabolism
   d. Feto-maternal haemorrhage
   e. Vitamin K deficiency

2. **What three investigations are indicated to help diagnosis?**
   a. Mother and baby blood group
   b. Coombs test
   c. Cranial ultrasound
   d. Bilirubin level
   e. Echocardiography
   f. Serum ammonia
   g. Kleihauer test
   h. G6PD level

Case 92

An 11-month-old Pakistani boy is referred with jaundice and pallor. His haematological investigations reveal:

Hb   4.3 g/dl
Plt $260 \times 10^9/l$
WCC $8 \times 10^9/l$ (normal differential)
Ret   9%
MCV   77 fl
MCHC   25 g/dl
Blood film No basophilic stippling

1. **What is the diagnosis?**
   a. β–thalassaemia
   b. Spherocytosis
   c. Iron deficiency anaemia
   d. Sickle cell anaemia
   e. None of the above

2. **How may this be confirmed?**
   a. Blood film
   b. Bone marrow aspiration
   c. Ferritin and iron-binding capacity level
   d. Hb electrophoresis
   e. Osmotic fragility test

3. **What is the management?**
   a. Splenectomy at age of 5 years
   b. Folic acid supplement
   c. Regular transfusion with SC desferrioxamine
   d. Oral iron supplement and dietician referral
   e. Bone marrow transplant
   f. Genetic counselling

Case 93

A 6-year-old Caucasian girl presents with abdominal pain. She is lethargic and slightly jaundiced with large spleen. She has not been ill recently, but a family member has required abdominal surgery for a similar problem. Her results were:

Hb   7 g/dl
MCHC   39 g/dl (34 g/dl)
Ret   13%
Plt   300 × 10⁹/l
WCC   6.4 × 10⁹/l

Blood film shows Howell–Jolly bodies, spherocytes, anisocytosis and megalocytosis

1. **What is the cause of her abdominal pain?**
   a. Splenomegaly
   b. Haemolytic crisis
   c. Gall bladder stone
   d. Gastric irritation
   e. Renal stone

2. **What is the most likely underlying diagnosis?**
   a. Biliary obstruction
   b. Acute cholecystitis
   c. Acute pancreatitis
   d. Spherocytosis
   e. Liver cirrhosis

3. **List two other useful tests to prove your diagnosis:**
   a. Hb electrophoresis
   b. Abdominal ultrasound
   c. Abdominal CT scan
   d. Blood film
   e. Serum amylase
   f. Osmotic fragility test
   g. Cholangiography
   h. Bone marrow biopsy

Case 94

An 11-year-old boy is found to be comatose. He is sweating profusely. His mother suffered a heart attack one year ago.

His blood gases are:

pH	7.07 kPa
Po_2	12 kPa in air
Pco_2	3.5 kPa
HCO^{-3}	12 kPa
BE	−12.3
Na	131 mmol/l
K	2.3 mmol/l
U	4.5 mmol/l
Cr	45 mmol/l
Albumin	35 mmol/l
Urine reducing substance	Positive
Glucose	7.8 mmol/l
CT	Normal

1. **Describe the blood gas result:**
    a. Respiratory acidosis
    b. Metabolic acidosis
    c. Respiratory alkalosis
    d. Metabolic alkalosis
    e. Compensatory respiratory acidosis

2. **What is the underlying diagnosis?**
    a. Inborn error of metabolism
    b. Drug intoxication
    c. Sepsis
    d. Asthma
    e. Renal failure

Case 95

A term infant is noticed to have extensive bruises over his lower limbs and chest at 8 hours of age. Further investigations show:

Hb	17.7 g/dl
WCC	$11 \times 10^9/l$ (L 70%)
Plt	$14 \times 10^9/l$
PTT	60 s (70–90)
PT	14 s (13–16)
TT	7 min

1. **List two differential diagnoses.**
    a. Isoimmune thrombocytopenia
    b. Sepsis
    c. Autoimmune thrombocytopenia – SLE
    d. ITP
    e. Von Willebrand disease

2. **Give one confirmatory test for each diagnosis**
    a. INR
    b. BT
    c. Blood film
    d. Platelet antibody level (baby and mother)
    e. Factor VIII level
    f. Factor X level
    g. Von Willebrand factor level
    h. rNP antibodies (baby and mother)

Case 96

At one hour of age, an infant is noted to be dusky and irritable. His weight is 4.7 kg. He is jittery, with a respiratory rate of 60. Investigations reveal:

Hb	25 g/dl
WCC	$15 \times 10^9/l$
Plt	$400 \times 10^9/l$
CRP	<5
PCV	77%
CXR	Normal
Arterial pH	7.34
Po_2	11 kPa
Pco_2	4.3 kPa
BE	−4.2

1. **What is the underlying problem?**
    a. Methaemoglobinaemia
    b. Polycythaemia
    c. Sepsis
    d. Neonatal abstinence syndrome
    e. None of the above

2. **What three steps would you choose for management?**
    a. Serial blood glucose
    b. Serial serum calcium level
    c. Partial exchange transfusion
    d. Nil per mouth
    e. 10 ml/kg of 0.9% saline as a bolus dose
    f. IV antibiotics
    g. Cranial ultrasound

Case 97

A 2½-year-old girl has normal motor developmental skills. She seems to be very shy. She plays alone and has no eye contact with others in the room. She has minimum understanding of verbal words. She can say >10 single words and no sentences. She plays repetitive games and builds a tower of 7 cubes.

1. What is the most likely diagnosis?

2. At what age is her language development?

Case 98

The following milk preparation was given to a 1-week-old infant.

Protein	3.8 g/100 ml
Fat	3.4 g/100 ml
CHO	4.4 g/100 ml
Na	1.44 mmol/100 ml
K	1.51 mmol/100 ml
Ca	2.8 mmol/100 ml
PO_4	1.6 mmol/100 ml

1. What type of milk is this?

2. Why is it not suitable for babies of 1 week of age?

Case 99

A 15-year-old boy emigrated from India. He has had a history of recurrent abdominal pain over the last year. His father is a doctor and his mother has terminal breast cancer. No abnormality is found on examination. He passes black stools every time that he defecates.

Hb	9.3 g/dl
WCC	$6.4 \times 10^9/l$
Na	139 mmol/l
K	4.3 mmol/l
ESR	25 mm/h
CXR	Normal
LFT and clotting	Normal
Abdominal US and X-ray	Normal
MSU	Normal

1. What is the most likely diagnosis?
   a. Gastritis
   b. GOR
   c. Intermittent malrotation
   d. Meckel diverticulum
   e. IBD

2. What simple test will you do to support your diagnosis?
   a. pH study
   b. Barium swallow
   c. Upper GIT endoscopy with biopsy
   d. ^{99m}Tc scan
   e. Abdominal MRI scan with contrast

3. **What is the treatment?**
   a. Nothing
   b. Referral to psychologist
   c. Proton pump inhibitors
   d. Steroids
   e. Laparotomy

Case 100

A 9-year-old girl presents with a history of progressive loss of vision and painful eyes. She has an area of numbness on her face. Fundoscopy reveals bilateral papilloedema. She becomes ataxic, and the MRI shows areas of demyelination in both cerebral hemispheres.

1. **What is the most likely diagnosis?**
   a. Multiple sclerosis
   b. Acute demyelinating encephalomyelitis (ADEM)
   c. Hysterical
   d. Optic neuritis
   e. Metachromatic leukodystrophy

2. **List three other investigations that may help in diagnosis.**
   a. CSF for oligoclonal bands
   b. MRI spine
   c. Very long-chain fatty acids (VLCFA)
   d. VEP
   e. EEG

3. **What treatments are available for this condition?**
   a. Corticosteroids
   b. IVIG
   c. Lumbo-peritoneal shunt
   d. Interferon-β
   e. Diuretics

Case 91

1. Feto-maternal haemorrhage
2. Direct Coombs test (DCT)
   Kleihauer test
   G6PD level

Feto-maternal haemorrhage

It is vital to look for evidence of haemolysis in a newborn baby less than 24 hours of age presenting with anaemia. All results can be obtained on the same day, apart from G6PD level.

Feto-maternal haemorrhage usually occurs spontaneously in the last trimester, with an increased rate during the first and second stages of labour. It may follow amniocentesis, fetal blood sampling, intrauterine transfusion and external cephalic version. How the fetal red blood cells get into the maternal circulation is still unknown. It can be identified by the Kleihauer test even if only 0.5 ml of fetal blood enters the maternal circulation.

This test depends on the fetal red blood cells resisting acidification at low pH while adult red blood cells lose their haemoglobin, leaving deeply pigmented fetal cells in a sea of maternal ghost cells. Feto-maternal haemorrhage rarely causes problems to the mother, but leaves a newborn baby anaemic.

Case 92

1. β–thalassaemia
2. Hb electrophoresis
3. Regular blood transfusion
   SC desferrioxamine
   Genetic counselling
   Bone marrow transplant

Haemoglobinopathy in children

Thalassaemia minor	HbF 20%, HbA$_2$ increase
Sickle cell anaemia	HbS deficiency
Sickle cell trait	HbAS
Thalassaemia major	HbF 90% and HbA$_2$ 10%

	Thalassaemia	Sickle cell anaemia
Aetiology	Imbalance in globin chain production	Substitution of valine for glutamine in position 6 of the β chain for HbS
Presentation	Before 1st birthday	After 6 months of age and rarely before 3 months of age
Haemoglobinopathy	*Thalassaemia major: HbF + A$_2$ HbF >90% HbA$_2$ 10% *Thalassaemia trait: HbA$_2$ + A$_1$ ± F	Sickle cell anaemia: HbS + F Sickle cell trait: HbS + A HbC and HbC trait
Inheritance	AR/D	AR
Crises	Haemolytic anaemia Splenomegaly Extramedullary haemopoiesis	Haemolytic Aplastic Sequestration Painful crises (hand–foot syndrome) Infarctions
Treatment	Regular transfusion Desferrioxamine (SC) Bone marrow transplant Folic acid	May need transfusions Regular folic acid Analgesia for crises/hydration Bone marrow transplant

Case 93

1. Splenomegaly
2. Spherocytosis
3. Osmotic fragility test
   Abdominal ultrasound

Spherocytosis

Spherocytosis is caused by a red cell membrane defect that causes a loss of surface area, and this is associated with the severity of the spherocytosis. Histochemical analysis shows a cytoskeletal protein defect in the red cell membrane. The spherocytic cell has increased osmotic fragility.

Causes

These include ABO incompatibility, thermal injuries, clostridial septicaemia, and Wilson disease.

Diagnosis

The fragility test, blood film and MCV are normal but the reticulocyte count is high and MCHC and bilirubin are increased.

Treatment

Transfusion can be given if Hb <10 g/dl, reticulocytes 10% and there is an aplastic crisis with splenomegaly. Splenectomy is carried out when the spleen is causing a lot of abdominal pain with frequent aplastic crises. It is preferable to delay this until the child is over 6 years old, if possible. Vaccination against *Haemophilus influenzae*, pneumococcus and meningococcus is indicated in all splenectomy patients.

Laboratory features and possible diagnosis in children with splenomegaly

Spherocytes on blood film, low haemoglobin, family history	Spherocytosis
Low haemoglobin, high HbA$_1$	Thalassaemia
Aplastic crises with sickle cells on blood film	Sickle cell anaemia
Anaemia, neutropenia, protozoa on blood film	Malaria, leishmaniasis
Abnormal liver function, positive hepatitis serology, stigmata of chronic hepatic failure, neutropenia, anaemia	Portal hypertension
Large vacuolated cells in bone marrow. Sphingomyelinase deficiency in leukocytes or fibroblasts, cherry red spot on retina in 25% of patients	Niemann–Pick disease A and B
Gaucher cells in bone marrow and reticuloendothelial system, β-glucocerebrosidase deficiency in leukocytes and fibroblasts	Gaucher disease type 1 (bony abnormalities, no CNS involvement) Gaucher disease type 3 (supranuclear horizontal ophthalmoplegia, CNS involvement)

Case 94

1. Metabolic acidosis
2. Drug intoxication

Salicylate poisoning

The pH is low with normal P_{O_2} and slightly low P_{CO_2}. This indicates a severe metabolic acidosis with mild respiratory alkalosis.

Pathophysiology

Salicylate is a respiratory stimulant, which leads to hyperventilation and respiratory alkalosis in the beginning. This is followed by metabolic acidosis. K and Na are both lost in urine with the bicarbonate. Despite this, the plasma Na and K are normal at this stage. When sufficient K has been lost, an exchange of K with H$^+$ occurs and the urine becomes acidic. This will cause a reduction of salicylate secretion in the urine. This aciduria occurs in the presence of respiratory alkalosis.

Dehydration, hypokalaemia and progressive accumulation of lactic acid will cause metabolic acidosis. The patient has rapid breathing at this stage because of metabolic acidosis rather than because of respiratory stimulation by salicylate. The patient may develop pulmonary oedema with 10–15% dehydration. Hypoprothrobinaemia may develop and the patient requires regular clotting screens.

Different features of acid–base balance:

	pH	P_{CO_2}	P_{O_2}	HCO^{-3}
Metabolic acidosis	Low	Normal	Low	Low
Respiratory acidosis	Low or normal	High	Low	High or normal
Metabolic alkalosis	High	High or normal	Low or normal	High
Respiratory alkalosis	High	Low	Low or normal	Low

Management

Correction of dehydration is very important, as is maintaining the patient's electrolytes. IV or IM vitamin K should be given. Hypo- or hyperglycaemia should be corrected; insulin can be used if necessary. Forced alkaline diuresis can be used in moderate and severe cases. Alkalization of the urine is the important thing rather than the induction of excessive urine flow. Peritoneal dialysis may be required in severe cases. Counselling is essential; the patient should be referred to a psychiatrist.

Differential diagnosis in cases most commonly presenting with metabolic acidosis (blood tests)

	Blood sugar	Blood pH	Lactate	Ammonia	Ketones
DKA	High	Low	Normal	Normal	High
Organic acidaemia	Low	Low	High	High or normal	High
Salicylate	High or low	High at beginning then low	Normal or low	Normal	Normal
Sepsis	High or low	Low	Low or high	Normal	Low
Lactic acidosis	Low	High	Normal	Normal	
Mitochondrial disorders	Normal or low	Low	High	Normal	Normal
Urea cycle defect	Normal	Low	Norma		Normal
Hyperglycinaemia	Normal	Normal	Normal	Normal	Normal

Case 95

1. Isoimmune neonatal thrombocytopenia (INT)
   Autoimmune – SLE mother
2. Platelet antibody (baby and mother)
   rNP antibodies (baby and mother)

Isoimmune neonatal thrombocytopenia (INT)

This follows transplacental transfer of maternal-specific IgG antiplatelet antibody from a platelet antigen-negative sensitized mother. This sensitization can occur at any time and can affect more than one newborn from the same mother.

Causes

Chronic maternal idiopathic thrombocytopenia, maternal SLE and drugs, e.g. isoniazid and sulphonamide, can produce INT.

Treatment

Options include corticosteroids, which show variable results. IVIG gives good results. If platelets are $<10 \times 10^9/l$, this is an indication for exchange transfusion followed by maternal washed platelet transfusion.

A list of possible causes of neonatal thrombocytopenia

Age	Most common aetiology	Less common aetiology
Fetal	1. Alloimmune 2. Congenital infection (e.g. CMV, toxoplasma, rubella) 3. Aneuploidy (e.g. trisomies 18, 13, 21, or triploidy) 4. Autoimmune (e.g. ITP, SLE)	1. Severe rhesus disease 2. Congenital/inherited (e.g. Wiskott–Aldrich syndrome)
Early onset neonatal (<72 h)	1. Placental insufficiency (e.g. gestational proteinuric hypertension (GPH), IUGR, diabetes) 2. Perinatal asphyxia 3. DIC 4. Alloimmune 5. Autoimmune	1. Congenital infection (e.g. CMV, toxoplasma, rubella) 2. Thrombosis (e.g. aortic, renal vein) 3. Bone marrow replacement (e.g. congenital leukaemia) 4. Kasabach–Merritt syndrome 5. Metabolic disease (e.g. propionic and methylmalonic acidaemia) 6. Congenital/inherited (e.g. thrombocytopenia and absent radius syndrome (TAR), congenital amegakaryocytic thrombocytopenia (CAMT))

| Late onset neonatal | 1. Late onset sepsis
2. NEC | 1. Congenital infection (e.g. CMV, toxoplasma, rubella)
2. Autoimmune
3. Kasabach–Merritt phenomenon
4. Metabolic disease (e.g. propionic and methylmalonic acidaemia)
5. Congenital/inherited (e.g. TAR, CAMT) |

Case 96

1.   Polycythaemia
2.   Serial blood glucose
     Serial serum calcium level
     Partial exchange transfusion if arterial PCV > 70% or PCV > 65% and symptomatic

Newborn polycythaemia

Newborn babies with polycythaemia look plethoric; central venous haematocrit is >0.65 or 0.70 from peripheral venous blood. It is necessary to do an arterial haematocrit if the baby is not symptomatic and Hct is >0.70 from venous blood. If the Hct from the arterial sample is <0.70 and the child is asymptomatic, there is no need to do an exchange transfusion. Exchange transfusion should be done with fresh frozen plasma, and Hct should come down to <50%.

Plasma volume required

$$= \frac{\text{estimated blood volume} \times \text{observed Hct} \times \text{desired Hct}}{\text{observed Hct}}$$

Causes

These include intrauterine hypoxia due to maternal diabetes, pre-eclampsia, maternal smoking, post maturity and growth retardation. An increase in erythropoietin level in infants with Down syndrome may cause polycythaemia.

Clinical features

The most common complications in infants with polycythaemia are renal vein thrombosis, bleeding because platelets are low, necrotizing enterocolitis, seizures and hyperbilirubinaemia. Infants are usually lethargic, not feeding well, and hypotonic.

Case 97

1. Autism (language and social developmental delay)
2. 15–18 months

Social dysfunction syndromes in children

Social dysfunction of various kinds is the main criterion for autism and Asperger syndrome.

	Autism	Asperger syndrome
Social dysfunction	Deficient in superficial social skills, empathy, compassion	Superficial social skills, empathy, compassion are impaired
IQ	Often low	Often normal or high
Onset	Before age of 30 months	At any age
Social interaction	Impaired (relationship, share, eye-to-eye contact)	Same as autism
Emotional reciprocity	Impaired	Impaired
Communication	Impaired	Not impaired
Language	Delayed	No clinically significant delay
Imaginative	Delayed	No delay
Ritual behaviour	Yes	Yes
Preoccupation	Yes	Yes
Stereotyped and repetitive motor	Yes	Yes
Mannerisms restricted	Yes	Yes
Cognitive	Delayed	No delay

Case 98

1. Cows' milk
2. High sodium, protein and phosphate

Infant formulas

Casein-dominant	Whey-dominant
Milumil	Aptamil
Cow & Gate Plus	Cow & Gate Premium
Farley's Second	Farley's First
SMA White	SMA Gold

Whey-dominant formula closely mimics the casein:whey ratio of breast milk. There is no difference between the two in terms of calorie content.

Casein-dominant formula has a slightly higher content of protein, sodium, potassium, calcium and phosphorus. Casein-dominant formulas have added carbohydrate.

Case 99

1. Gastritis
2. Upper GIT endoscopy
3. Proton pump inhibitors

Recurrent abdominal pain

This is one of the common paediatric problems occurring in older children and adolescents. The pain is usually non-specific and has been described as colicky, periumbilical discomfort, varying in duration, not radiating or altered by position or daily activity. There are other organic causes that need to be ruled out. Patients with peptic ulceration or gastritis have pain, usually radiating to the back, which wakes them at night, and a strong family history; the condition may be associated with iron deficiency anaemia. Food intolerance may cause recurrent abdominal pain, and elimination of certain foodstuffs may help. Migraine may also cause recurrent abdominal pain; there is a family history and response to anti-migraine drugs. Urinary tract infection and renal calculus have to be ruled out. There are also other suggestions that recurrent abdominal pain may be due to alteration in gastrointestinal motility. Constipation can cause this problem, and a full bowel history and examination may exclude it. Abdominal X-ray is helpful but should not be routine.

Other causes that need to be looked for include inflammatory bowel disease, pancreatitis, hepatobiliary disease, and anatomical abnormalities (malrotation, Meckel diverticulum). Selective laboratory and radiological tests with full history and examination will help to find out what the problem is.

Case 100

1. Multiple sclerosis
2. CSF for oligoclonal bands
   MRI spine
   Visual evoked potentials (VEP), somatosensory evoked response (SSER)
3. Corticosteroids
   Interferon-β

Demyelinating diseases in children

	Clinical	Neuroimaging	Neurophysiology
Multiple sclerosis	Optic neuritis Sensory disturbances Diplopia Ataxia	Cranial CT may show areas of low density MRI: increased signals on T2-weighted sequence of white matter in both hemispheres	VEP and SSER increase in latency BSAER decrease in amplitude of wave V Oligoclonal banding present in 85% of patients
Acute demyelinating encephalomyelitis (ADEM)	Multifocal CNS disturbances Drowsiness or coma, seizures	MRI: increased signals on T2 of both white and grey matter	VEP, SSER and BSAER are normal Oligoclonal banding is normal
Optic neuritis	Sudden mono- or bilateral visual impairment Neuropapillitis	MRI: increased signals on T2 of one or both optic nerves	VEP increases in latency SSER and BSAER are normal Intrathecal IgG oligoclonal production increased
Acute transverse myelitis	History of acute infection in 60% Acute pain and paraplegia Sphincter and sensory disturbances	MRI: increased signals on T2 of spinal cord	VEP and BSAER are normal NCS is abnormal EMG is normal Meningitis, SLE, vascular abnormalities should be excluded

With permission from Gerald M Fenichel (WB Saunders)

Neuromyelitis optica, Schilder myelinoclastic diffuse sclerosis and AIDS myelopathy are rare in children and should be excluded.

Corticosteroids are effective in the treatment of all demyelinating diseases of childhood; duration and mode of administration vary according to the condition.

EMQs

From the following scenarios, choose the most appropriate diagnosis from List A and the two most appropriate investigations that may help in the diagnosis from List B.

Case 101

A 7-month-old boy presents with continuous seizures and requires ventilation. He looks dysmorphic, with sparse hair, low-set ears and VUR on MCUG.

Blood gas
pH	7.35
P_{CO_2}	4.7 kPa
HCO^{-3}	17 kPa
BE	−1
Ammonia	35 mmol/l
Lactate	1.2 mmol/l
Amino acids	Normal
VLCFA	Normal
Glucose	4.5 mmol/l
Urates	1.2 mmol/l
Copper	Low
Caeruloplasmin	Low
MRI brain	Old subdural collection, generalized brain atrophy

Skeletal survey shows generalized osteoporosis

Case 102

A 9-month-old boy presents with a history of myoclonic jerks controlled by clobazam and global developmental delay. His parents are consanguineous.

Blood gas
pH	7.33
P_{CO_2}	4.4 kPa
HCO^{-3}	16 kPa
BE	−0
Ammonia	80 mmol/l
Lactate	4.3 mmol/l
Amino acids	N
VLCFA	N
Glucose	3.5 mmol/l
Urates	1.2 mmol/l
CSF lactate	3.5 mmol/l
CSF glucose	2.5 mmo/l

MRI brain   Generalized brain atrophy
EMG and NCS   Normal reading

Case 103

A 10-day-old baby presents with vomiting and lethargy and is sleepy.

Blood gas:
pH   7.21
P_{CO_2} 5.7 kPa
HCO^{-3} 13 kPa
BE   −12
Blood:
Ammonia   1500 mmol/l
Lactate   1.2 mmol/l
Amino acids   Normal
VLCFA   Normal
Glucose   4.5 mmol/l
Urates   1.2 mmol/l
MRI brain   No abnormalities

Case 104

A 6-year-old girl presents with a history of seizures, which happened twice in the early morning. They lasted for 2 minutes and then she was very sleepy.

Blood gas:
pH   7.34
P_{CO_2} 4.5 kPa
HCO^{-3} 18 kPa
BE   −2
Ammonia   60 mmol/l
Lactate   1.2 mmol/l
Amino acids   Normal
VLCFA   Normal
Glucose   1.5 mmol/l
Urates   1.2 mmol/l
Carnitine   High

Case 105

A 3-month-old boy presents with a history of lethargy, not feeding and being jittery.

Blood gas:
pH   7.32
P_{CO_2} 4.3 kPa
HCO^{-3} 16 kPa

BE	–5
Ammonia	70 mmol/l
Lactate	1.4 mmol/l
VLCFA	Normal
Isotransferrin	Normal
Glucose	4.5 mmol/l
Urates	1.2 mmol/l
Amino acids	Abnormal (high alanine, low phenylalanine and taurine)
Urine organic acids	Normal
MRI brain	Generalized brain atrophy

List A

a. Urea cycle defect
b. Propionic acidaemia
c. Mitochondrial disorders
d. Phenylketonuria
e. Menkes syndrome
f. Carbohydrate glycoprotein deficiency
g. Wilson disease
h. Beta-oxidation defect of fatty acid
i. Non-ketotic hyperglycinaemia
j. Fructosaemia
k. Tyrosinaemia

List B

a. Urine organic acid
b. White cell enzymes
c. Acyl carnitine level
d. Skin biopsy for tissue fibroblasts
e. Liver biopsy
f. CSF lactate
g. VLCFA
h. Hair for microscopic study
i. MRI brain
j. Molecular genetic study
k. Blood gas
l. Blood glucose
m. Urine amino acid

EMQs

From the following scenarios, choose the most likely diagnosis from List A and match it with the most appropriate treatment(s) from List B.

Case 106

A 14-year-old girl is brought to Casualty by her parents with a history of hyperventilation, difficulty in breathing and pyrexia. She is very sleepy. She had an argument with her mother this morning before she went to school and is otherwise a healthy young girl.

Blood gas:

pH	7.51
P_{CO_2}	2.5 kPa
P_{O_2}	9.8 kPa
HCO^{-3}	13
BE	12
Lactate	2.7 mmol/l
Glucose	3.0 mmol/l

Urine for reducing substances is positive; no other drugs

Case 107

A 10-year-old boy and his mother are brought to A&E with a history of shortness of breath, headache, dizziness and vomiting. Gas maintenance work where the family live was done two weeks ago.

Blood gas:

pH	7.29
P_{CO_2}	2.5 kPa
HCO^{-3}	13 kPa
BE	−6
P_{O_2}	9.8 kPa
Lactate	2.7 mmol/l
Glucose	3.0 mmol/l

Case 108

A 5-week-old boy presents with a history of vomiting, which his mother says can reach the other end of the room.

Blood gas:

pH	7.49
P_{CO_2}	4.5 kPa
HCO^{-3}	22 kPa
BE	2
P_{O_2}	8.0 kPa
Lactate	1.7 mmol/l
Glucose	4.0 mmol/l

Case 109

A 25-day-old female baby presents with jaundice. She is the first child of non-consanguineous parents. She has been breastfed from day one.

Hb	15.5 g/dl
CRP	<5 mg/l (0–8)
WCC	$8 \times 10^9/l$
Total bilirubin	175 µmol/l (0–23)
Conjugated bilirubin	66 mmol/l
Plt	220×10^9
ALP	290 u/l (109–272)
ALT	20 u/l (0–45)
MCV	70 fl
MCHC	90 fl
PT	13 s
APTT	120 s
INR	1.6
Serum α_1-antitrypsin	Normal
Sweat test	Cl <40 mmol/l

Abdominal ultrasound shows absence of the gallbladder with no dilatation of the biliary tree

Case 110

A 13-year-old girl presents with joint pain and swelling, mild fever up to 38 °C and tiredness.

Hb	9.5 g/dl
CRP	<15 mg/l (0–8)
WCC	8×10^9 (N 2.7, L 5.1, E 1.0, M 0.5, B 0.0)
Total bilirubin	11 µmol/l (0–23)
ALP	300 u/l (109–272)
ALT	20 u/l (0–45)
Plt	$550 \times 10^9/l$
ANA	Positive
DNA double-strand	Negative
Urine analysis	No red or white cells

Synovial biopsy shows synovial infiltration with plasma cells, mature B lymphocytes, and T lymphocytes, with areas of synovial thickening and fibrosis

List A

a. Systemic lupus erythematosus
b. Hypothyroidism
c. Choledochal cyst
d. Bacterial endocarditis
e. Biliary atresia
f. Paracetamol toxicity
g. Galactosaemia

h. Neonatal cholestasis
i. Carbon monoxide poisoning
j. Reiter syndrome
k. Juvenile chronic arthritis
l. Salicylate toxicity
m. Hepatitis B
n. Pyloric stenosis

List B

a. Haemodialysis
b. Kasai procedure
c. IV antibiotics
d. Peritoneal dialysis
e. IV Parvlex
f. Pyloromyotomy
g. Gastric lavage
h. Oral activated charcoal
i. Oral thyroxine
j. Oral steroids
k. Ursodeoxycholic acid
l. Galactose-restricted diet
m. Hyperoxygenation
n. Sodium bicarbonate
o. NSAID
p. Methotrexate

Case 101

1. Menkes syndrome
2. Molecular genetic study
   Hair for microscopic study

Menkes syndrome

Menkes syndrome is an X-linked recessive disorder characterized by generalized copper deficiency. Mutations in the *ATP7A* gene are associated with Menkes syndrome. It is characterized by kinked hair, growth retardation, severe neurological problems including seizures, and global developmental delay. There are also renal abnormalities, with hydronephrosis and nephropathy. Changes in the metaphyses of the long bones and tortuosity of cerebral arteries have been described. Hypothermia and acute illness with septicaemia are modes of presentation. There is patchy abnormality of the systemic arteries, with stenosis or obliteration. The syndrome is also associated with hypotonia, low-set ears and white skin, even in non-white families.

Some of the tests that may be done include:

- X-ray of the skeleton or X-ray of the skull
- Serum copper level
- Skin cell (fibroblast) culture
- Serum caeruloplasmin

Death occurs within the first or second year of life.

Case 102

1. Mitochondrial disorders
2. White cell enzymes
   Skin biopsy for tissue fibroblasts

Mitochondrial disorders

An initial blood test should be done for suspected mitochondrial disorders.

Laboratory evaluation of mitochondrial disorders

- Lactate and pyruvate from blood (always high)
- Lactate/pyruvate ratio:
  - High (>50:1): suggests metabolic block in respiratory chain
  - Normal: metabolic block, which could be, e.g., pyruvate dehydrogenase complex (normal values do not exclude mitochondrial disorders).

- Serum CK:
  - Usually normal or mildly elevated
  - Could be high in chronic progressive external ophthalmoplegia (CPEO) and ptosis, limb weakness, or very high in mitochondrial DNA depletion
- Muscle biopsy: good for respiratory chain problems and muscle histology
- Skin biopsy for tissue fibroblasts for enzymatic assay
- Neuroradiology:
  - Bilateral signal intensities in putamen, globus pallidus and caudate (Leigh's disease)
  - Stroke-like lesions in posterior cerebral hemisphere (mitochondrial encephalopathy, lactic acidosis and stroke-like episodes: MELAS)
  - Diffuse signal change in central white matter (Kearns–Sayre disease)
  - Basal ganglia calcifications (Kearns–Sayre disease or MELAS)
- Molecular genetic mutation screening can be done in some cases, e.g. MELAS, MERRF (myoclonic epilepsy associated with ragged-red fibres).

Case 103

1. Urea cycle defect
2. White cell enzymes
   Skin biopsy for tissue fibroblasts

Urea cycle defect

The most likely diagnosis in this case is a urea cycle defect due to ornithine transcarbamylase (OTC) deficiency. Male patients usually present in the first few days of life with an encephalopathy-like illness and die after a few days if appropriate treatment is not given. It is an X-linked dominant disorder.

Female carriers may have a mild form of the disease. The onset occurs during high protein intake, infection or starvation. Death may occur following a coma with hyperammonaemia. Mental development is usually normal. There is a marked increase of urine orotic acid, which differentiates OTC from other forms of urea cycle defect.

The management of hyperammonaemia associated with urea cycle defects is as follows. Management of acute hyperammonaemia is with low protein (0.25 g/kg/day); phenylacetate, sodium benzoate and arginine should be given as soon as possible, and if there is no improvement then dialysis should be considered. If there is a good result, then maintain the above regimen. All patients should be supplied with an emergency kit for acute hyperammonaemia treatment.

Case 104

1. Fatty oxidation defect
2. VLCFA
    Acyl carnitine level

Fatty oxidation defect (FOD)

This is a disorder of mitochondrial fat oxidation. It is associated with one or all of hypoketotic hypoglycaemia, cardiomyopathy and cytopathy. The presentation of these children to a clinician could be as Reye-like syndrome, cardiomyopathy, hypotonia and developmental delay, hypoglycaemia, as well, in some cases, sudden infant death.

Tests that enable the clinician to diagnose suspected FOD are:

*   Plasma carnitine levels
*   Acyl carnitine profiles
*   Molecular tests

Urine tests that will help in diagnosis are:

*   Carnitine levels
*   Organic acids
*   Acyl carnitine profiles
*   Acyl glycine analysis

Skin biopsy (tissue fibroblasts) can be examined, looking for defects in any of these enzymes, and various other tests include:

*   Oxidation rates of C1 substrates
*   Tritium release assays using palmitate and myristate
*   In vitro probe of fat oxidation pathway
*   Specific enzyme or uptake assay
*   Mutation analysis

Case 105

1. Phenylketonuria
2. White cell enzymes (for PKU)
    Urinary amino acids

Phenylketonuria (PKU)

This is an inborn error of protein metabolism in which the essential amino acid phenylalanine will not metabolize. The serum level of phenylalanine will exceed 1200 mmol/l if treatment is not applied very soon. Patients with PKU may present with mental retardation unless levels of phenylalanine are controlled with a strict diet.

Screening and diagnosis of phenylketonuria

Newborn screening identifies almost every case of PKU. It is usually done on a Guthrie card within two or three days following birth, before the baby leaves the hospital. The baby must be fed and have some protein given before testing. Testing is done all over the UK as well as in many other developed countries. If the patient is proved to have PKU or suspected PKU, then a blood test must be done to confirm the diagnosis. Genetic testing to identify gene mutations can also be done. It is possible to detect PKU in a developing fetus using chorionic villus sampling (CVS).

Case 106

1.   Salicylate poisoning
2.   Oral activated charcoal

Salicylate poisoning

The pH is low with normal Po_2 and slightly low Pco_2. This indicates a severe metabolic acidosis with mild respiratory alkalosis.

Pathophysiology

Salicylate is a respiratory stimulant, which leads to hyperventilation and respiratory alkalosis in the beginning. This is followed by metabolic acidosis. K and Na are both lost in urine with the bicarbonate. Despite this, the plasma Na and K are normal at this stage. When sufficient K has been lost, an exchange of K with H^+ occurs and the urine becomes acidic. This will cause a reduction of salicylate secretion in the urine. This aciduria occurs in the presence of respiratory alkalosis.

Dehydration, hypokalaemia and progressive accumulation of lactic acid will cause metabolic acidosis. The patient has rapid breathing at this stage because of metabolic acidosis rather than because of respiratory stimulation by salicylate. The patient may develop pulmonary oedema with 10–15% dehydration. Hypoprothrobinaemia may develop and the patient requires regular clotting screens.

Management

Correction of dehydration is very important, as is maintaining the patient's electrolytes. IV or IM vitamin K should be given. Hypo- or hyperglycaemia should be corrected; insulin can be used if necessary. Forced alkaline diuresis can be used in moderate and severe cases. Alkalization of the urine is the important thing rather than the induction of excessive urine flow. Peritoneal dialysis may be required in severe cases. Counselling is essential; the patient should be referred to a psychiatrist.

Differential diagnosis in cases most commonly presenting with meta-bolic acidosis (blood tests)

	Blood sugar	Blood pH	Lactate	Ammonia	Ketones
DKA	High	Low	Normal	Normal	High
Organic acidaemia	Low	Low	High	High or normal	High
Salicylate	High or low	High at beginning then low	Normal or low	Normal	Normal
Sepsis	High or low	Low	Low or high	Normal	Low
Lactic acidosis	Low	High	Normal	Normal	
Mitochond-rial disorders	Normal or low	Low	High	Normal	Normal
Urea cycle defect	Normal	Low	Normal		Normal
Hyper-glycinaemia	Normal	Normal Normal	Normal	Normal	

Case 107

1. Carbon monoxide poisoning
2. Hyperoxygenation

Carbon monoxide poisoning

Symptoms

Exposure to carbon monoxide (CO) can be associated with the following symptoms: headache, dizziness, nausea, fainting, seizure, flu-like symp-toms, shortness of breath on exertion, impaired judgement, chest pain, depression, hallucinations, agitation, fatigue, vomiting, abdominal pain, drowsiness, visual changes and confusion.

Management

1. Remove the patient from the area of high CO.
2. Take the patient to hospital and give oxygen en route to hospital.
3. Identify the source of CO.
4. The most effective treatment for CO poisoning is high-dose oxygen, usually using a facemask attached to an oxygen reserve bag.
5. In severe poisoning, a hyperbaric pressure chamber may be used to give even higher doses of oxygen.

Case 108

1. Pyloric stenosis
2. Pyloromyotomy

Hypertrophic pyloric stenosis

The history is very important in the clinical diagnosis of pyloric stenosis. The child usually presents during the 2nd–4th weeks of life, sometimes later (4th month). The usual story is of projectile vomiting, but not all projectile vomiting is due to pyloric stenosis. A history of vomiting shooting to the other side of the room or dining table is quite suggestive.

The feeding test is very important. Use either the index, middle or ring finger of your left hand to palpate the upper quadrant of the abdomen during feeding. You need to be on your knees on the left side of the infant. This is an important test, and is almost diagnostic as it will reveal a pyloric 'tumour'.

Abdominal ultrasound is a complementary test and provides reassurance that the diagnosis is correct. Another criterion is hypochloraemic alkalosis with signs of dehydration. Peristaltic movement can also be observed during feeding, moving from left to right.

Treatment

First, correct dehydration by IV fluid – 5% glucose and 0.9% saline, adding KCl.

Pyloromyotomy (Ramstedt operation) is the surgical treatment. Oral feeding can be started 24 hours after surgery.

Case 109

1. Biliary atresia
2. Kasai procedure

Biliary atresia

Investigations

- Start with liver function tests and proceed to more invasive tests for diagnostic purposes.
- Liver enzymes are high (ALT, AST, ALP), there is conjugated hyperbilirubinaemia, low albumin and total protein, and abnormal prothrombin time and partial thromboplastin time (PTT).
- Viral titres to exclude hepatitis A, C, B and HIV.
- Blood culture to exclude bacterial infection.
- Abdominal ultrasound.
- Hepatobiliary scan (HIDA).
- Liver biopsy is the most definitive diagnostic test.

Treatment

There is no medication that will help. Supportive treatment should be given as soon as the diagnosis is made and until surgery takes place, preferably before the infant is 60 days old. A Kasai portoenterostomy connects the bile drainage from the liver directly to the intestinal tract. It is most successful when done before an infant is 8 weeks old. The Kasai procedure is helpful so that the child can grow normally. Up to 80% of children who undergo Kasai portoenterostomy will eventually require a liver transplant.

Case 110

1. Juvenile chronic arthritis (JCA)
2. Methotrexate (MTX)

Juvenile chronic arthritis

Juvenile chronic arthritis (JCA) is a group of diseases associated with single or multiple joint involvement. The cause is not known. The disease is characterized by chronic inflammation of synovium, which is caused by B lymphocyte infiltration and expansion. There are several types of JCA, including systemic onset, pauciarticular and polyarticular.

The ESR is elevated, there may be lymphopenia, thrombocytopenia and normocytic, normochromic anaemia. Antinuclear antibody (ANA) is observed in as many as 25% of children with JCA, especially in children with pauciarticular disease. If found to be high in young girls, it may indicate an increased risk of uveitis or other diseases such as SLE.

Rheumatoid factor is high in adults with polyarticular JCA.

A multidisciplinary team approach should be adopted when treating children with JCA. Medication initially includes NSAIDs, which can be given in all types of JCA. Naproxen is commonly used. Aspirin should not be used for children under 12 years of age.

The second choice is methotrexate, which is an immunosuppressive agent. It is useful and effective in children with polyarticular JCA and some with aggressive pauciarticular disease. Other drugs include sulfasalazine, methylprednisolone and prednisone.

The third option is to use etanercept, which is a tumour necrosis factor (TNF) inhibitor. TNF is but one of many cytokines involved in the inflammatory cascade that contributes to the symptoms associated with JCA.

EMQs

From the following scenarios, choose the most appropriate diagnosis from List A and match it with two further treatments from List B.

Case 111

A 75-day-old baby who was born at 27 weeks' gestation has required two transfusions since birth. He is pale and lethargic and has developed apnoea. A full septic screen was done and he has been treated for two days with IV antibiotics. All cultures showed no growth.

Hb	6.5 g/dl
CRP	<5 mg/l (0–8)
WCC	8 × 10⁹/l
Total bilirubin	11 µmol/l (0–23)
ALP	300 u/l (109–272)
Plt	190 × 10⁹/l
ALT	17 u/l (0–45)
MCV	70
MCHC	70
Hct	<1
ESR	<10

Blood film shows no abnormalities

Case 112

The following results are from a term baby with a history of pallor, oedema and no booking of blood during pregnancy. The parents have just migrated to this country and have received no antenatal care.

Blood film shows nucleated RBC, reticulocytosis, polychromasia, aniso-cytosis, 60% spherocytes and cell fragmentation.

Blood taken at age of 4 hours:

Hb	14.0 g/dl
CRP	<5 mg/l (0–8)
WCC	8 × 10⁹/l (N 3.7, L 4.1)
Plt	170 × 10⁹/l
Total bilirubin	40 µmol/l (0–23)
ALP	160 u/l (109–272)
ALT	15 u/l (0–45)
MCV	70 fl
MCHC	90 fl
PCV	41%
Direct Coombs test	Weakly positive

Case 113

A baby girl was born at 34 weeks' gestation with APGAR 4@1 and 5@3 and 8@10.

Her mother has had three miscarriages and one healthy child aged 3 years.

Hb	17.0 g/dl
CRP	40 mg/l (0–8)
WCC	13 × 10⁹/l (N 6.7, L 6.1)
Total bilirubin	20 μmol/l (0–23)
ALP	190 u/l (109–272)
ALT	14 u/l (0–45)
Plt	130 × 10⁹/l
MCV	77 fl
MCHC	90 fl
PCV	55%

Blood culture after 24 hours showed Gram-positive cocci

Case 114

A 24-hour-old baby boy was born at term without any difficulties. He has become jittery and irritable, and is not feeding well.

Hb	21.0 g/dl
CRP	<5 mg/l (0–8)
WCC	8 × 10⁹/l (N 3.7, L 4.1)
Plt	170 × 10⁹/l
Total bilirubin	10 μmol/l (0–23)
ALP	180 u/l (109–272)
ALT	18 u/l (0–45)
MCV	72 fl
MCHC	95 fl
PCV	70%
Glucose	4.5 mmol/l
Blood film	Polychromasia

Case 115

A 3-day-old baby girl is admitted to the neonatal unit with a history of irritability, high-pitched cry, excessive sweating and hyperreflexia. There was no antenatal care. The mother is known to have hepatitis B and another child in foster care.

Hb	16.0 g/dl
WCC	11 × 10⁹/l
ALP	140 u/l (109–272)
ALT	16 u/l (0–45)
Plt	190 × 10⁹/l

CRP	<5 mg/l (0–8)
Total bilirubin	7 μmol/l (0–23)
Glucose	4.1 mmol/l
Ca	2.13 mmol/l
Mg	0.85 mmol/l

List A

a. Infant of diabetic mother
b. Necrotizing enterocolitis
c. Polycythaemia
d. Hypoglycaemia
e. Neonatal sepsis
f. Group B streptococcal sepsis
g. ABO incompatibility
h. Hydrops fetalis
i. Neonatal abstinence syndrome
j. Anaemia of prematurity
k. Metabolic bone disease of prematurity
l. Inborn error of metabolism
m. Hepatitis B

List B

a. Partial exchange transfusion
b. IV penicillin and gentamicin
c. Oral morphine sulphate
d. Blood transfusion
e. Ventilatory support if needed
f. Iron supplement
g. Chloral hydrate at night
h. Maintain hydration
i. Triple phototherapy
j. Vitamin D supplement
k. Total exchange transfusion
l. Sodium feredetate (Sytron)
m. Folic acid

EMQs

Choose from the following scenarios the most appropriate diagnosis from List A and match it with one diagnostic test from List B that will support your diagnosis.

Case 116

A 10-day-old baby girl presents with a history of lethargy, not feeding well and vomiting.

Plasma concentrations:

Pregnenolone	High
17-hydroxypregnenolone	High
DHEA	High
17-hydroxyprogesterone (17-OHP)	High
Cortisol	Low
Aldosterone	Low
Androstenedione	Low
ACTH	High
Follicle-stimulating hormone (FSH)	High
Luteinizing hormone (LH)	High

Case 117

A 2-year-old girl presented with breast tissue and sparse pubic hair.

Oestradiol	20 pg/ml
Dehydroepiandrosterone (DHEA)	High
Dehydroepiandrosterone sulphate (DHEAS)	High
17-OHP	Within normal range
LH	0.1 IU/l
FSH	1.7 IU/l
T$_4$	19 IU/l

Case 118

A 10-year-old boy presents with headache, flushing and generalized muscle weakness. His blood pressure is 130/80 mmHg.

Na	138 mmol/l
K	3.1 mmol/l
U	1.4 mmol/l
Cr	50 mmol/l
Albumin	45 mmol/l
Total protein	66 mmol/l
ALP	180 mmol/l
ALT	32 mmol/l
Urine	No proteinuria or blood

Case 119

A 4-year-old girl presents with abdominal pain, nausea and generalized muscle weakness.

Na	136 mmol/l
K	4.1 mmol/l
U	1.4 mmo/l
Cr	55 mmol/l
Ca	2.76 mmol/l
Albumin	39 mmol/l
Total protein	70 mmol/l
ALP	350 mmol/l
ALT	30 mmol/l
P	1.1 mmol/l

Bone density on X-ray is very low in all the vertebrae and other bones.

After exercise test:

GH	<4 ng/l (>7)
Cortisol	170 mIU/l (<200)
FSH and LH	Prepubertal
TSH	1.8 mIU/l (<5)

Case 120

A 6-month-old child presented with a history of constipation, hypotonia, hoarse cry and jaundice. There were also coarse facial features.

Na	136 mmol/l
K	4.1 mmol/l
U	2.3 mo/l
Cr	60 mmol/l
Albumin	44 mmol/l
Total protein	70 mmol/l
ALP	160 mmol/l
ALT	25 mmol/l
Urine	No proteinuria or blood
TSH	50 mIU/l
T$_4$	9.1 mIU/l
Cortisol	180 mIU/l
Testosterone	<1 mIU/l

List A

a. Hypothyroidism
b. Hyperaldosteronism
c. 3β-Hydroxysteroid dehydrogenase
d. Growth hormone deficiency
e. Pseudo-precocious puberty
f. Congenital adrenal hyperplasia
g. Precocious puberty
h. Nelson disease
i. Hyperparathyroidism
j. Hypophosphataemic rickets

List B

a. Glucagon stimulation test
b. GnRH test
c. Insulin suppression test
d. Thyroid iodine scan
e. Pelvic ultrasound
f. Abdominal CT
g. Abdominal MRI
h. Urinary 17-hydroxypregnenolone

Case 111

1. Anaemia of prematurity
2. Sodium feredetate (Sytron)
   Folic acid

Anaemia of prematurity

The most common pathophysiology of anaemia of prematurity is failure of the immature kidney to secrete erythropoietin as the PCV and Hb fall below the normal range. As a result of this, the bone marrow is not stimulated, which results in failure to produce enough red cells. Other causes of anaemia in newborn babies include:

- Infection (e.g. septicaemia and syphilis)
- Repeated removal of small volumes of blood for special investigations (e.g. blood gases)
- Haemolytic disease of the newborn
- Haemorrhage before delivery (feto-maternal haemorrhage)
- Haemorrhage at or after delivery (e.g. bleeding from the umbilical cord)

Iron deficiency does not cause anaemia in the newborn period, but iron supplements should be given to all premature babies from the age of 28 days up to 6 months. If iron supplement is not given early, then iron deficiency anaemia is common after 3 months in all premature babies.

Case 112

1. ABO incompatibility
2. Triple phototherapy
   Maintain hydration

ABO incompatibility

ABO haemolytic disease occurs if the mother is blood group O and her fetus is blood group A or B. The fetus usually inherits these blood groups from the father. ABO haemolytic disease is the most common cause of severe jaundice in term infants. The haemolysis is not as severe as in rhesus disease and will not damage the fetus, but may cause severe jaundice in the newborn infant. ABO haemolytic disease may occur in both early and late pregnancy.

The maternal antibodies, which stick to the fetal red cells, give a mild to moderate positive Coombs test in the newborn infant, while the haemolysis results in a low packed cell volume and haemoglobin. This will lead to raised total serum bilirubin within the first 24 hours. The baby is usually born normal and no jaundice is detected in the first few hours after birth. The baby will develop anaemia, and it is important to introduce phototherapy early. Very rarely, the baby will need exchange transfusion and may need blood transfusion if the haemoglobin drops to the lowest level. Maintaining hydration with feed or IV fluids is very important. Unfortunately ABO haemolytic disease is not preventable, nor can it be diagnosed accurately before delivery.

Case 113

1. Group B streptococcal sepsis
2. High dose of IV ampicillin and gentamicin
   Ventilatory support if needed

Group B streptococcal sepsis

It is thought that 10–30% of women in the UK carry group B strepto-coccus (GBS) in the vagina. Certain groups of babies are at high risk of developing GBS septicaemia:

- The mother has had a previous baby infected with GBS.
- The mother has had a vaginal swab confirming GBS colonization in the current or previous pregnancies.
- The mother has had GBS bacteruria at any time in the current preg-nancy.
- Preterm, premature rupture of membranes with or without signs of labour.
- Preterm labour and delivery before 35 completed weeks' gestation.
- The mother has had a fever >38 °C during labour.
- Prolonged rupture of membranes >24 hours.

GBS is the leading cause of neonatal septicaemia all over the world. Major risk factors include those listed above and low levels of maternal serum anti-GBS antibodies. Early onset of this disease can be prevented by screening for maternal GBS colonization. Late-onset GBS disease is unlikely to be reduced by these strategies. The other strategy is to give prophylactic antibiotics during labour to all mothers who are colonized with GBS to reduce the risk of GBS in their babies.

Case 114

1. Polycythaemia
2. Partial exchange transfusion
   Maintain hydration

Polycythaemia

Polycythaemia can be defined as a packed cell volume (PCV) above 65%. It is important that the blood is venous, arterial or capillary blood taken with clear flows so that PCV can be measured accurately. The baby appears plethoric and asymptomatic in most cases. Symptomatic babies may present with neurological signs, respiratory distress, hypoglycaemia or heart failure.

The causes of polycythaemia are:

- Intrauterine growth restriction (IUGR)
- Infant of diabetic mother
- Twin to twin transfusion
- Delayed cord clamping.

Non-symptomatic polycythaemia does not need treatment. The baby can be fed early and hydration should be maintained at all times. If the baby becomes symptomatic or PCV > 75%, then partial plasma exchange transfusion can be carried out using either normal saline or fresh frozen plasma not exceeding 20 ml/kg. It is similar to the exchange transfusion method, and the baby should be kept warm all the time.

Case 115

1. Neonatal abstinence syndrome
2. Oral morphine sulphate
   Chloral hydrate at night

Neonatal abstinence syndrome

This syndrome is the result of symptoms and signs occurring in the infant of an opioid-dependent woman. It is characterized by signs and symptoms of the central nervous system: hyperirritability (which may lead to convulsions), gastrointestinal dysfunction (diarrhoea), sweating and hunger, respiratory distress and vague autonomic symptoms that include yawning, sneezing, mottling and fever.

A multidisciplinary team approach should be adopted in these cases and a plan of action should be in place before the baby is delivered. The mother should be screened for infectious diseases, including HIV. Her nutritional status should be monitored, and any other risk factors should be considered.

Social services, the GP and health visitor should be informed and a case conference should be held as soon as the baby is born.

The baby should be monitored in the neonatal unit with 4-hourly observations. No baby should be given naloxone after birth, as it will cause respiratory arrest.

If the baby becomes symptomatic, withdrawal symptoms should be controlled with morphine or Oramorph as per the protocol. Seizures should be stopped by loading with phenobarbital and keeping the baby on a maintenance dose. Feeding should be guided according to the weight of the baby, as these are usually hungry babies. Most symptoms start to appear 72 hours after birth.

When discharged, care should be planned with the mother, and social services will go with the mother or to the foster carer. Follow-up should be undertaken as needed.

Case 116

1. Congenital adrenal hyperplasia
2. Urinary 17-hydroxypregnenolone

Congenital adrenal hyperplasia (CAH)

The commonest enzyme deficiency associated with CAH is 21-hydroxylase deficiency.

Clinical features

Newborn male infants commonly do not show any abnormality (occasionally a Caucasian newborn will have a dark scrotum). Newborn female infants show virilization as a result of exposure to DHEA, testosterone and aldosterone. Female infants are usually born with ambiguous genitalia. They may present with salt-loss crisis by the age of 3–4 weeks. Salt-loss crises can occur in both male and female infants.

Investigation of ambiguous genitalia

Test	Comment
Karyotype	Preliminary results available within 48 hours
17-OHP in plasma or blood spot	Placental 17-OHP may interfere in first 24 hours Overlap with the raised levels in sick or preterm infants is rare
Electrolytes:	
Plasma K	Increased. Often precedes fall in Na
Plasma Na	Decreased
Urinary Na	Increased
Plasma testosterone	Frequently within adult male range
Plasma renin activity (PRA)	Increased. Sensitive index of salt depletion, but result seldom available immediately
Urinary steroid metabolites	Confirms site of block, especially in the rare enzyme defects
Pelvic ultrasound	Reassures parents about normal female internal genitalia
Sinogram	Occasionally required to show internal genital anatomy

Permission has been granted by Professor Ieuan A Hughes to use this material

Cloning of the gene by DNA analysis can be done to determine carrier status as well as enabling prenatal diagnosis to be carried out.

In girls, surgical correction can be done at the age of puberty.

Approximately 5% of CAH is due to 11β-hydroxylase deficiency. These cases can present similarly to 21-hydroxylase deficiency but with high blood pressure.

Treatment

Cortisol replacement (hydrocortisone 12–25 mg/m²/day in two doses) is given. It is necessary to monitor growth and virilization as well as 17-OHP and testosterone levels. Patients also require salt and aldosterone replacement (salt – up to 5 mmol/kg/day; fludrocortisone).

Case 117

1. Pseudo-precocious puberty
2. Pelvic ultrasound

Pseudo-precocious puberty

In pseudo-precocious puberty, high levels of testosterone or oestrogens are produced by a tumour or other abnormality in the adrenal gland or in a testis or ovary. These hormones do not cause the testes or ovaries themselves to mature but do cause a child to look more like an adult. Pubic and underarm hair grows, adult body odour develops, and the child's body shape changes. Acne may also appear.

The cause could be isolated premature thelarche. There is evidence of increased oestrogen production and high basal GnRH-stimulated FSH levels. Pelvic ultrasound may show ovarian cysts with a moderately enlarged uterus.

Adrenarche may present as pubic and/or axillary hair growth with increased height velocity and breast enlargement or enlarged testes. CAH is the commonest cause; Cushing syndrome and adrenocortical tumours are other possible causes.

Gonadal causes such as testicular or ovarian tumours may also cause pseudo-precocious puberty, as may ingestion of sex steroids (oestrogen, mainly either by the pregnant mother or via contaminated food).

Case 118

1. Hyperaldosteronism
2. Glucagon stimulation test

Hyperaldosteronism

In hyperaldosteronism, there is overproduction of aldosterone, which can lead to fluid retention and increased blood pressure, weakness and, rarely, periods of paralysis due to low potassium.

Aldosterone, a hormone produced and secreted by the adrenal glands, stimulates the kidneys to excrete less sodium and more potassium. Aldosterone production is regulated partly by corticotropin and partly through the renin–angiotensin–aldosterone system. Renin is an enzyme produced in the kidneys that controls the activation of the hormone angiotensin. Angiotensin stimulates the adrenal glands to produce aldosterone.

177

Hyperaldosteronism can be caused by a tumour – usually a non-malignant adenoma in the adrenal gland (Conn syndrome). There can be unilateral or bilateral gland involvement. Sometimes, hyperaldosteronism may be a response to certain diseases, such as very high blood pressure or narrowing of one of the renal arteries.

If a tumour is found, this should be removed surgically. The blood pressure will return to normal, and other symptoms should disappear. If no tumour is found, and both glands are overactive, partial removal of the adrenal glands may not control high blood pressure, and complete removal will produce Addison disease, requiring treatment for life. If there has been partial removal, and blood pressure remains high and potassium is low, then spironolactone can usually control the symptoms, along with other drugs for high blood pressure.

Case 119

1. Growth hormone deficiency
2. Glucagon stimulation test

Growth hormone deficiency/insufficiency (GHD/GHI)

The incidence is 1 in 4000 and the aetiology is varied. GHD/GHI may be congenital or acquired. Congenital causes are:

- Genetic (types IA, B, II and III) GHRH receptor gene mutation
- Brain abnormalities (septo-optic dysplasia, holoprosencephaly, encephalocele, hydrocephalus and agenesis of corpus callosum)
- Idiopathic.

Acquired causes include trauma, meningitis/encephalitis, craniopharyngioma, histiocytosis, pituitary germinoma and cranial irradiation. GHD/GHI may also be transient (psychosocial deprivation, hypothyroidism and per pubertal).

Short stature and poor height velocity are the two types of presentation. An older child with GHD/GHI may have an immature face with prominent forehead, midfacial hypoplasia, increased subcutaneous fat, delayed dentition, delayed bone age and micropenis. The hypothalamic–pituitary axis should be investigated after exclusion of other causes. Bone age can be done early, as well as karyotyping.

Indications for use of growth hormone

- Children with severe GHI/GHD.
- Moderate GHI.
- Girls with Turner syndrome may be benefit from GH.
- Children with extreme IUGR who remain short may benefit from GH.
- Skeletal dysplasia (not much benefit).
- GHRH therapy may be appropriate in many problems that are hypothalamic in origin rather than pituitary.

Case 120

1. Hypothyroidism
2. Thyroid iodine scan

Hypothyroidism

The causes include:

1. Agenesis of the thyroid gland
2. Inflammation of the thyroid gland (Hashimoto thyroiditis)
3. Treatment of hyperactive thyroid (surgery or radioactive therapy)
4. Panhypopituitarism

The patient may present with fatigue; weakness; weight gain or increased difficulty losing weight; coarse, dry hair; dry, rough pale skin; hair loss; cold intolerance; muscle cramps and frequent muscle aches; constipation; depression; irritability; memory loss; and abnormal menstrual cycles.

Hashimoto thyroiditis (also called autoimmune or chronic lymphocytic thyroiditis) is the most common type of thyroiditis. The thyroid gland is always enlarged, but this may be unilateral. The thyroid gland cells have failed and are unable to convert iodine into thyroid hormone, so the gland 'compensates' by enlarging. This will mean that the uptake of radioactive iodine is high while the patient is hypothyroid, because the gland retains the ability to take up or 'trap' iodine even after it has lost its ability to produce thyroid hormone. As the gland becomes less able to function, the TSH increases since the pituitary is trying to induce the thyroid to make more hormone; the T_4 falls since the thyroid is unable to produce it. So, the thyroid function test will show high TSH and low T_4. Thyroid antibodies are present in 95% of patients with Hashimoto thyroiditis and serve as a useful marker without the need for thyroid biopsy or surgery.

Treatment is to start thyroid hormone replacement. The patient should be monitored with thyroid function tests on a regular basis until the correct dose has been established and thyroid function normalized. In most cases, the thyroid gland will decrease in size once thyroid hormone replacement is instigated. Thyroid antibodies may remain for years even after successful treatment.

De Quervain thyroiditis (also called subacute or granulomatous thyroiditis) is the second most common thyroiditis and much less common than Hashimoto thyroiditis. The thyroid gland usually swells very rapidly and becomes very painful and tender. The gland releases thyroid hormone into the blood and patients become hyperthyroid; however, the gland will stop taking up iodine and this problem will resolve in a few weeks. Patients frequently become ill with fever and lethargy. The ESR is high and thyroid antibodies are not present in the blood. There is no need for antibiotics; they are ineffective and the thyroiditis will resolve spontaneously. Analgesia and bed rest will help to overcome this problem. Sometimes, thyroxine can be given to rest the gland along with steroids for any inflammation. This combined treatment should be given over short periods, 2–3 weeks only. Rarely, some patients become hypothyroid once the inflammation settles down, and will therefore need to stay on thyroid hormone replacement indefinitely.

Silent thyroiditis is the third and least common type of thyroiditis. It is similar to De Quervain thyroiditis, but there is no pain and needle biopsy resembles Hashimoto thyroiditis. No treatment is required and 80% of patients show complete recovery and return of the thyroid gland to normal after 3 months. Symptoms are similar to Graves disease except that they are milder. The thyroid gland is only slightly enlarged and exophthalmos does not occur. Treatment is usually bed rest with beta-blockers to control palpitations.

EMQs

From the following scenarios, choose the most likely diagnosis from List A and match it with one more investigation from List B to help in diagnosis.

Case 121

A 3-month-old girl presents with history of floppiness, inability to suck and lethargy. Reflexes are absent in the upper and lower limbs.

CSF:
WCC   11/mm^3
RBC   30/mm^3
Glucose   3.4 mmol/l
Protein   2.8 mmol/l (0.6–8)
Gram stain   Negative
Culture   Negative after 48 hours

Head and spine MRI scan with gadolinium show increased signals in the lumbar regions (L2–5).

Case 122

A 7-year-old girl presents with proximal muscle weakness. She is having difficulty standing from a sitting position.

CK   500 mmol/l
ESR   <10mm/h

Muscle biopsy shows fibre necrosis, fatty replacement and excessive collagen. The nerve conduction study is normal as is MRI of the brain and spine.

Case 123

A 10-day-old child presents with a history of being unwell, lethargic and starting to have focal seizures on the right.

CSF:
WCC   60/mm^3 (70% lymphocytes)
RBC   37/mm^3
Glucose   3.1 mmol/l
Protein   0.7 mmol/l (0.6–8)
Gram stain   Negative
Culture   Negative after 48 hours
Blood glucose 5.3 mmol/l
CRP   15 mg/l
EEG shows wave activities, no focal discharges

Case 124

A 7-year-old child presents with a history of ataxia, dysarthria, dysphonia and inability to swallow liquid food. Power, tone and reflexes in the upper and lower limbs are entirely normal. CSF shows no abnormalities. PCR for HSV is negative.

Case 125

A 10-year-old girl presents with abnormal movements in her arms and legs, which look like spasms, occurring 10–20 times per hour.

CSF:
WCC   1/mm^3
RBC   5/mm^3
Glucose   3.4 mmol/l
Protein   0.5 mmol/l (0.6–8)
Gram stain   Negative
Culture   Negative after 48 hours
Lactate   5.1 mmol/l (<1.2)
Blood glucose 5.3 mmol/l
CRP   10 mg/l
Lactate   8.1 mmol/l (2–2.3 mmol/l)
Serum amino acids and urine organic acids reports as normal
MRI of spine and brain shows white matter changes

List A

a. Wilson disease
b. Meningoencephalitis
c. Transverse encephalomyelitis
d. Acute disseminated encephalomyelitis
e. TB meningitis
f. Myopathy
g. Encephalitis
h. Bulbar palsy
i. Mitochondrial disorders
j. Infantile spasms
k. Myoclonic epilepsy
l. Lennox–Gastaut syndrome
m. Severe myoclonic epilepsy of infancy
n. Multiple sclerosis
o. Barbiturate poisoning
p. Aseptic meningitis

List B

a. Cranial MRI scan with gadolinium
b. Nerve conduction study of cranial nerves IX and XII
c. White cell enzymes
d. Molecular genetic study for severe myoclonic epilepsy of infancy (SMI) gene
e. Skin biopsy
f. Caeruloplasmin level
g. EEG
h. Electromyography
i. CSF PCR for HSV
j. CSF PCR for mycobacteria
k. Wood light test
l. Cranial CT
m. CSF IgG oligoclonal bands
n. Nerve conduction study

Case 121

1. Transverse encephalomyelitis
2. Nerve conduction study

Transverse encephalomyelitis

This is an acute inflammation of the spinal cord that evolves in hours or days. It affects teenagers and older age groups. It may be associated with demyelination of the CNS. It may follow infectious illness or immunization, but there is no supportive evidence for this. There are both motor and sensory signs and the thorax is the usual level of myelitis. Asymmetrical leg weakness is common. There is a bladder-emptying problem, with increased or reduced tendon reflexes in the lower limbs. Recovery usually starts after a week and may be incomplete. Fifty per cent will recover completely, 40% will recover incompletely, and 10% will not recover. MRI of the spine shows cord compression and swelling at the level of the myelitis. CSF shows raised white cells and elevated IgG. Corticosteroids are used in treatment: high-dose IV for 3 days followed by a minimum of 4 weeks oral. The bladder problem may require rehabilitation and involvement of the urologist and specialist nurse.

Case 122

1. Myopathy
2. EMG

Proximal muscle weakness

Proximal muscle weakness is most often caused by different myopathies. Juvenile spinal muscular atrophy is the only one that can cause proximal muscle weakness, and EMG and muscle biopsy will distinguish it from myopathy.

Other causes are myasthenia syndromes, muscular dystrophies, inflammatory myopathies (dermatomyositis and polymyositis), metabolic myopathies (acid maltase deficiency, carnitine deficiency, lipid storage myopathies and mitochondrial myopathies) and endocrine myopathies (adrenal cortex, parathyroid and thyroid diseases).

Differentiation between proximal weakness

	Myopathy	Neuropathy	Myasthenia
Tendon reflexes	Depressed or absent	Absent	Present
EMG	Amplitude, brief, small polyphasic motor unit	Fasciculations, high denervation amplitude polyphasic motor unit	Normal
Nerve conduction studies	Normal	Normal or mildly slow	Abnormal repetitive stimulation
CK	High	Normal	Normal
Muscle biopsy	Fatty fibre necrosis, replacement of excessive collagen	Group atrophy, group typing	Normal

Case 123

1. Aseptic meningitis
2. CSF PCR for HSV

Aseptic meningitis

This is usually caused by drugs or a virus. Viral meningitis is self-limiting and recovery occurs in >95% of patients. Patients usually present with abrupt high temperature, headache and stiff neck, except for infants, who usually have a bulging fontanelle. Irritability, lethargy and vomiting are common. The CSF will show 10–200 leukocytes/mm^3 (mainly lymphocytes), protein 0.5–1.0 g/l, and normal glucose concentration.

CSF should be sent for HSV PCR if herpes infection is suspected and the meningitis treated accordingly. The infant or child will recover within one week from aseptic meningitis, although some may continue to experience headache and tiredness. There is no need to check hearing. Bed rest, analgesia and maintaining hydration is the treatment for aseptic meningitis.

Case 124

1. Bulbar palsy
2. Cranial MRI and MRA

Bulbar palsy

	Bulbar palsy	Pseudobulbar palsy
Cranial nerves	XII–VII	Corticobulbar tracts
Presentation	Lips – tremulous speech	Tongue – paralysed, no wasting initially and no fasciculation; 'Donald Duck' speech; unable to protrude
	Tongue – weak and wasted and sits in the mouth with fasciculation	
	Drooling – as saliva collects in the mouth and the patient is unable to swallow (dysphagia)	Palatal movements absent Persistent dribbling
		Facial muscles – may also be paralysed
	Palatal movements absent Dysphonia – rasping tone due to vocal cord paralysis; nasal tone if bilateral palatal paralysis	Reflexes – exaggerated, e.g. jaw jerk
		Nasal regurgitation may be present
	Articulation – difficulty pronouncing *r*; unable to pronounce consonants as dysarthria progresses	Dysphonic
		Dysphagic
		Emotional lability may also be present
Causes	Diphtheria	Cerebrovascular events, e.g. bilateral internal capsule infarcts
	Poliomyelitis	Demyelinating disorders (MS)
	Motor neurone diseases, e.g. progressive bulbar palsy	Motor neurone disease
	Cerebrovascular events of the brainstem	High brainstem tumours
		Horner syndrome Syringobulbia – look for nystagmus
	After radiotherapy for nasopharyngeal carcinoma or acoustic neuroma	Guillain–Barré syndrome
		Head injury
		Poliomyelitis
		Neurosyphilis
Investigations	MRI and CT	Cranial MRI and CT
	Also according to cause	Also according to cause
Treatment	Depends on the cause	Depends on the cause
	Supportive with multi-disciplinary team	Supportive with multi-disciplinary team
Prognosis	Depends on the cause	Depends on the cause

Case 125

1. Acute disseminated encephalomyelitis
2. CSF oligoclonal bands

Acute disseminated encephalomyelitis (ADEM)

ADEM usually follows a viral illness or measles immunization. In some cases, no cause can be found. It is a form of autoimmune phenomenon. The symptoms can be abrupt or insidious. Abrupt onset may consist of loss of consciousness and seizures. With insidious onset, there may be pyramidal or extrapyramidal signs, ataxia, facial palsy and nystagmus, or other forms of presentation. The CSF shows pleocytosis and a mild increase in protein. IgG oligoclonal band testing should be done to differentiate ADEM from other demyelinating disorders such as MS. MRI will show increased signals on T2-weighted images, usually involving the white matter. Spinal cord lesions are clearly seen, and may enhance with gadolinium.

Treatment is usually supportive if the diaphragm and bulbar nerves are involved. Corticosteroids (3 days IV and 3 weeks oral) are the treatment for this condition, and more than 70% of patients will recover.